Fibromyalgia: Pain Management:

Nutritional Healing For Pain Relief From Back Pain, Chronic Pain, Nerve Pain to Pain Free for Life

Mia Soleil

Fibromyalgia Book Guide

How to Successfully Live with Fibromyalgia and Recipes for the Fibromyalgia Diet

Mia Soleil

Image courtesy of photostock at FreeDigitalPhotos.net

© Copyright 2014 by Joy Publishing & Marketing Corporation - All rights reserved.

This document is geared towards providing helpful and reliable information in regards to the topic and issue covered. The publication is sold with the idea that the publisher is not required to render accounting, officially permitted, or otherwise, qualified services. If advice is necessary, legal or professional, a practiced individual in the profession should be ordered.

- From a Declaration of Principles which was accepted and approved equally by a Committee of the American Bar Association and a Committee of Publishers and Associations.

In no way is it legal to reproduce, duplicate, or transmit any part of this document in either electronic means or in printed format. Recording of this publication is strictly prohibited and any storage of this document is not allowed unless with written permission from the publisher. All rights reserved.

The information provided herein is stated to be truthful and consistent, in that any liability, in terms of inattention or otherwise, by any usage or abuse of any policies, processes, or directions contained within is the solitary and utter responsibility of the recipient reader. Under no circumstances will any legal responsibility or blame be held against the publisher for any reparation, damages, or monetary loss due to the information herein, either directly or indirectly.

Respective authors own all copyrights not held by the publisher.

The information herein is offered for informational purposes solely, and is universal as so. The presentation of the information is without contract or any type of guarantee assurance.

The trademarks that are used are without any consent, and the publication of the trademark is without permission or backing by the trademark owner. All trademarks and brands within this book are for clarifying purposes only and are the owned by the owners themselves, not affiliated with this document.

Table of Contents

Introduction   1

Chapter 1 – Dealing with Fibromyalgia   3

Chapter 2 – Treatments and Other Ways to Stop
Fibromyalgia from Ruining Your Life   11

Chapter 3 – Lifestyle Change for Fibromyalgia
Sufferers   15

Chapter 4 – Exercises that Can Help Alleviate the
Symptoms of Fibromyalgia   19

Chapter 5 – Sugar: The Sweet Poison at the
Root of It All   23

Chapter 6 – Alkaline or Acidic?   29

Chapter 7 – The Power of Hydration   31

Chapter 8 – Recommended Fibromyalgia Diet: Foods to
Eat and to Avoid   35

Chapter 9 – Recipes to Try   45

Conclusion   61

Preview Of Next Book   63

Introduction

I want to thank you and congratulate you for purchasing the book, *"Fibromyalgia Book Guide: How to Successfully Live with Fibromyalgia and Recipes for the Fibromyalgia Diet."*

This book contains treatments, strategies and recipes on how to successfully live with fibromyalgia and manage your pain.

Fibromyalgia is a chronic condition that influences more than 5 million people, a large majority being women. The constant pain and fatigue from fibromyalgia robs the individual from enjoying everyday life. Trying to find ways to manage and cope with this disorder can be very taxing to those who are affected by it.

I, too, have suffered from chronic pain and have felt its daily debilitating effects. I know the frustration of living a life packed with medical appointments, aggravation, discouragement and hopelessness. Fibromyalgia can be ruthless, unrelenting and difficult to conquer however things can turn around for the better.

My desire for you is to find encouragement and relief from your fibromyalgia through this book. I hope you will find treatments and lifestyle adjustments that you can make in your everyday life to help rein in this beast. Take heart, there is hope. Be strong. Preserve, pursue and fight for a life at peace with fibromyalgia.

I wish you luck on your path to wellness. To help you achieve the better version of yourself, I and my colleagues at Joy Publishing invite you to like our Facebook Page: www.facebook.com/joypublishing. Get free books and know of our new releases by joining us.

I sincerely thank you again for purchasing this book. I truly hope you enjoy it! Please take some time to stop by and LIKE our Facebook page:

https://www.facebook.com/joypublishing

With gratitude,

Mia Soleil

Chapter 1 - Dealing with Fibromyalgia

Fibromyalgia is classified as a non-threatening, chronic disorder. It is associated with a widespread pain in the musculoskeletal system accompanied with mood, stress, fatigue and sleep issues. It must be understood that fibromyalgia is not considered a disease, but a syndrome. It won't threaten your life, but the pain may become unbearable at any given time.

Most sufferers describe the condition as having persistent flu-like symptoms with pain being felt all over the body. The pain that it causes can be so severe that it has been linked to many cases of anxiety, headaches and even depression.

Although there is no scientific proof yet that having a proper diet and doing healthy lifestyle changes can indeed alleviate the symptoms of fibromyalgia, sufferers of the condition who chose to do modifications to their lifestyle and diet have seen significant improvement. If it worked for them, it will certainly do anyone suffering from the condition some good too, including you.

The Pain Is Not Just in Your Head

Because fibromyalgia is practically invisible, meaning x-rays or most lab tests do not and cannot give measurable findings regarding the condition, it does not mean that the pain you feel is just in your head. The pain is indeed real. The pain may not have any ability to inflict damage on the organs of your body or your joints but the relentless experience of being in pain can leave a significant influence in dealing with daily life.

The pain that comes with fibromyalgia can be so intense but without medical tests that can confirm it some sufferers are convinced that the pain they feel is only in their heads and that there is really no actual body pain. They think that their brain is just playing a nasty trick on them.

Currently, the medical community acknowledges the fact that the pain that is associated with having fibromyalgia is real. According to a research, it may be caused by a glitch in the manner that the body perceives or senses the pain. The researchers believe that the condition intensifies the pain sensation by influencing the processing of pain signals in the brain.

The symptoms sometimes start after a major psychological stress, surgery, physical trauma or infection. There are also cases where symptoms slowly progress within a certain period of time with an unknown trigger.

Risk Factors and Complications

Women are more likely to have fibromyalgia than men and it is also possible to develop it if someone in your family has the condition too. Individuals with lupus or rheumatoid arthritis and other rheumatic diseases are also more likely to have fibromyalgia.

Several individuals who have fibromyalgia also experience having temporomandibular joint (TMJ) disorders, tension headaches, depression, anxiety and irritable bowel syndrome (IBS).

Fibromyalgia can also lead to other problems and may make life even more difficult. The pain and lack of good sleep due to fibromyalgia can no doubt impede your ability to function properly at work or at home. The frustrations of handling the often misunderstood condition can lead to health-related anxiety and depression.

Today, there is still no known cure for fibromyalgia, but there are available medications that can help alleviate the symptoms and let you go through the day without so much trouble. Good diet, exercise, stress-reduction procedures, rest and relaxation may also help in improving the symptoms of this condition.

It is best to take necessary measures and start practicing a healthy lifestyle if you are someone who is at risk in developing the condition or has the condition already. Eating a well-balanced diet, avoiding certain foods, having a regular workout routine and maintaining a stress-free life can help a lot in keeping your condition under control.

Symptoms of Fibromyalgia

The most typical symptom of fibromyalgia is a widespread pain (the sufferer experiences pain on both sides of the body, as well as above and below the waist) which usually lasts for at least three months. There are cases wherein pain literally becomes a typical occurrence in the daily life of the victim. The pain can disturb the day to day existence of its victims especially those with a low pain threshold.

Sufferers of fibromyalgia often wake up in the morning feeling sluggish and tired even though they slept for many hours during the night. Their sleep is often interrupted by pain; in fact, several fibromyalgia victims also have sleep disorders like sleep apnea and restless legs syndrome.

Many individuals who suffer from fibromyalgia may also have constant headaches and cramps in the lower abdomen. There also exists a symptom that is typically referred to as "fibro fog" which impairs the ability of those with fibromyalgia to focus and concentrate on the work at hand.

Possible Causes of Fibromyalgia

Medical experts are still baffled regarding the real culprits or causes of fibromyalgia, but it is suspected that several factors that come together make the pain as intense as it is.

It is suspected that fibromyalgia may be an inherited condition. Scientific studies have been investigating genetic mutations or genetic markers that may be present in those who have fibromyalgia and their families.

There are also other conditions that may trigger the occurrence of fibromyalgia or make it much worse. Some experts believe that post-traumatic stress disorder (PTSD) can be one of the triggers the disease.

Women and Fibromyalgia

Around 80% to 90% of people diagnosed with fibromyalgia are women. The reason for such number may have something to do with the genes, hormones and differences in the immune system between the two sexes. Still, researchers are not exactly sure why women have the greater number of fibromyalgia sufferers than men.

Women who suffer from fibromyalgia often describe their pain as a dull ache that begins in the muscles. Sufferers experience pain on both sides of the body which also affects the upper and lower body parts. The pain can usually come and go for a period of at least three months. In some days, the pain can be so severe that it makes it impossible for a woman to stick with the planned activities for the day.

Many women with fibromyalgia have trouble keeping their focus and remembering things. They often mix up words when they talk or get confused more quickly than normal. These problems are collectively referred to as "fibro fog" because their minds feel foggy. Medical researchers are not quite certain regarding the cause of fibro fog, but they suspect that the lack of sleep or the effects on the brain of fibromyalgial pain may be the ones causing it.

Moreover, around half of fibromyalgia sufferers develop headaches. Several women get a throbbing headache or a migraine which can cause vomiting and nausea. The reasons for such an occurrence of headaches in fibromyalgia patients are still a mystery. Experts believe that the imbalance of chemicals in the brain, such as epinephrine and serotonin, may be the cause of the recurrent headaches.

One bodily system greatly affected in women with fibromyalgia is the reproductive system. One common symptom present in patients with fibromyalgia is menstrual cramps. These menstrual cramps can be extremely painful or just mild. Not all women experience these camps, but most women with fibromyalgia have more painful menstrual periods than normal. Some women with fibromyalgia also develop endometriosis in which the tissue from the uterus extends in some parts of the pelvis. Another problem that females with fibromyalgia experience is dyspareunia or painful sexual intercourse.

The digestive system is also affected by fibromyalgia. Irritable bowel syndrome or IBS is common in women who have fibromyalgia. IBS is characterized by symptoms like bloating, diarrhea, constipation and stomach cramps. Researchers are yet to discover the real reason behind the connection between IBS and fibromyalgia.

Sensitivity is another issue that most women with fibromyalgia must face. Most women who developed such sensitivity may find themselves grabbing their sweater whenever the temperature drops or experience profuse sweating when the temperature suddenly shoots up. Some women with fibromyalgia are also sensitive to bright lights and/or loud noises.

Tender Points

Aside from the widespread pain, fibromyalgia also creates tender points all over the body. These points are about as small as pennies and are called as such because they hurt when someone presses on them. You may feel the pain in some or all of the identified tender points.

These are all the possible tender points in the body:

- above the nape

- front portion of the neck

- area between the shoulders

- top portion of the chest (specifically, on the second rib)

- elbows

- upper portion of the buttocks

- hips

- insides of both knees

If you are in a lot of pain, it is possible that you have developed fibromyalgia. Although the evidence and facts regarding this dreadful condition can send shivers to the bones, it is still reassuring to know that it is not life-threatening. It could hinder you from giving out your best, but there are ways to alleviate the symptoms and still finish the task at hand without so much trouble. Make sure you seek professional help if you are suspicious of having fibromyalgia. This simple test using tender points is not a complete diagnosis and doctors can do much more to know and identify what disorder you are having.

Chapter 2 - Treatments and Other Ways to Stop Fibromyalgia from Ruining Your Life

Fibromyalgia sufferers can make the symptoms go away or at least lessen the severity of the symptoms with nutritious food, lifestyle changes and exercise. Studies reveal that enhanced physical fitness and having a certain diet can help alleviate the symptoms of fibromyalgia.

Therapy, acupuncture, counseling, pain medications and massage are also some of the things that may help sufferers in making the condition less debilitating.

Tests and Diagnosis for Fibromyalgia

Today, physicians can diagnose that a person is suffering from fibromyalgia based on where the pain is felt and how long it has been going on.

There is no laboratory test that can prove that a person has the condition, but through many diagnostic tests the doctor can rule out other possible conditions that have the same symptoms as fibromyalgia. The tests may involve, but not limited to, thyroid function tests, x-rays and blood tests.

Preparing for a Doctor's Appointment

Due to the several similarities of fibromyalgia with other conditions, the patient may need to see not just one doctor. The patient's family doctor may recommend or refer the patient to

11

doctors with different specializations since the pain is felt in many parts of the body and may involve different bodily systems.

It is best to prepare a detailed journal of the symptoms, the list of foods taken, habits, work, usual sleep patterns or if there's some trouble sleeping. Changes observed in the present and a detailed medical history can help a lot in the early diagnosis of fibromyalgia. The patient also needs to prepare his family medical history, as well as medications and supplements that he has taken or is currently taking. It is also best that the patient prepare a list questions or clarifications that the he wants to ask the doctor before the actual visit.

Common Treatments and Medications

Not all treatments and medications may work for all fibromyalgia victims, but a healthy diet and exercise can improve the condition of anyone.

There are patients who rely on pain relievers such as acetaminophen, naproxen sodium or ibuprofen to alleviate the pain. Some doctors may even give a prescription pain reliever for severe cases. However, taking narcotics is not a wise move to make because it can lead to dependence on the said drugs and may also cause worsening of the pain.

Antidepressants may be prescribed to help ease the fatigue and pain associated with fibromyalgia and also to aid the patients in getting restful sleep.

Anti-seizure medications, commonly used to treat epilepsy, may also be prescribed to help reduce some of the pain. Gabapentin and pregabalin are two popular anti-seizure drugs that can help reduce the symptoms of fibromyalgia in some patients.

Therapy and Alternative Medicine

Therapy and alternative medicine may work with some fibromyalgia patients. Some individuals attest that their condition improved when they tried a certain therapy or alternative medicine although these claims lack scientific evidence and still need further study.

One of the oldest methods that health care providers still practice today is massage therapy. This therapy involves using different techniques in manipulating the muscles and soft tissues of the body. Massage can definitely relax the muscles, bring down the heart rate and relax the nerves. It can also enhance the joints' range of motion, as well as increase the production of the natural painkillers of the body. It can effectively relieve anxiety and stress if done properly.

One type of massage, craniosacral therapy or CST, is a massage therapy which targets specific pressure points on the head and neck. Researchers discovered that those who had craniosacral massage therapy reported experiencing less pain and anxiety after a few sessions. Traces of depression had also diminished and they saw significant improvements in doing daily activities.

Another method called Cognitive Behavioral Therapy or CBT may also help fibromyalgia patients. CBT helps fibromyalgia patients identify negative thought patterns and turn them into something useful or beneficial to them. Researchers in Spain who evaluated fibromyalgia sufferers who went through the said therapy and some with combined hypnosis found out that the patients improved and that their symptoms were relieved faster as compared to using medications or drugs for their treatment.

Acupuncture, an ancient practice that originated in China, is also used by some to help alleviate the symptoms of fibromyalgia. It aims to restore the normal balance of life forces through the use of fine needles. These fine needles are inserted through the skin in varying depths. Western theories believe that the needles in acupuncture are responsible for changing the flow of blood and the neurotransmitter levels in the spinal cord and in the brain. The science behind how it works is not fully understood. The question of if it does indeed work has not been verified either.

Other forms of therapy like yoga and tai chi may also help control the symptoms of fibromyalgia. The practices combine slow movements, meditation, relaxation, and deep breathing.

These treatments may help alleviate the symptoms of fibromyalgia, but the relief they provide may only be temporary. Some drugs may even inflict more harm to the body in the long run especially if they are not monitored by health providers. Lifestyle changes, dietary modification and exercise may still prove to be the most effective solutions in battling its symptoms.

Chapter 3 - Lifestyle Change for Fibromyalgia Sufferers

In order to win against fibromyalgia, it is necessary to make some lifestyle adjustments that will help the sufferer in easing the pain, if not making all of it go away.

Eat Healthy Foods

Eating a well balanced diet can help a lot in alleviating the symptoms of fibromyalgia. It is a known fact that the body has the ability to heal itself by providing it with all the right nutrients and vitamins that the cells need in order to fight off harmful diseases or conditions.

Find Ways to Reduce Stress

Finding some means to reduce stress may seem next to impossible especially if there is constant pain, but there are ways to minimize or even eliminate stress in your life. Careful planning is the key in reducing stress. Work out a plan that will limit emotional stress and overexertion by setting a time each day to enjoy utmost relaxation.

Completely changing daily routines to get some much needed relaxation is necessary. Stressful activities may be removed or lessened in order to give more time for a little bit of R&R. Make your daily activities predictable but enjoyable to lessen the stress. If you know what will happen next, you will feel less distraught since you know what to expect. Stress management techniques such as meditation, deep breathing and getting massages may also help in relieving stress.

Adequate Sleep Is Important

Fatigue is one of the symptoms of fibromyalgia, that's why getting adequate sleep is fundamental in keeping all the symptoms at bay. Aside from setting ample sleeping time, practicing good sleeping habits like going to bed at the same time each night and waking up at the same time each morning can help a lot. It is also best to limit daytime naps to get sounder sleep at night. Watching TV or working on the computer should be discontinued at least 2 hours before going to sleep.

Keep A Regular Exercise Schedule

During the first few times, exercise may add to the bodily pain but doing the routine on a regular basis may soon decrease the symptoms of fibromyalgia. Exercises may include walking, biking and swimming. A physical therapist can also help the patient develop a simple exercise program at home.

Learn Pacing

It is equally important to keep activities on equal levels each day. Patients with fibromyalgia must be warned that doing too much on "good" days (where pain seems to be completely out of the picture) may yield more "bad" days in the future. A fibromyalgia sufferer must keep everything in moderation - meaning avoid overdoing things during the days when pain is less and almost doing nothing during the bad days when symptoms are at their worst.

Keep everything balanced by doing the work in exactly the same pace in all of the days regardless if a particular day is good or not. Again, do your best to keep all of your activities within schedule and establish a daily routine regardless of how you're feeling.

Maintaining a healthy lifestyle is not only good for fibromyalgia relief, but the overall health as well. People with fibromyalgia will be able to do away with drugs and other medications in the long run just by keeping a healthy lifestyle.

Chapter 4 - Exercises That Can Help Alleviate the Symptoms of Fibromyalgia

There are different exercises that can help ease the symptoms of fibromyalgia and make life easier for the sufferers. Many doctors suggest implementing a fitness or exercise program before considering any kind of medications or drugs. Even if the doctor prescribes a certain drug for the condition, staying active can play a huge role in making the pain go away.

How Much Exercise?

Some research show that having a workout for at least two times a week with a minimum of 25 minutes per session can yield significant improvement of the symptoms. It is prudent to start off with a low-to-moderate set of exercises like walking, water aerobics, swimming, biking, tai chi or yoga. Start slow then gradually increase the time and intensity of the exercise to a point that is still tolerable. Individuals with fibromyalgia must remember that it is imperative that they do not to overexert.

Warm up before working out. Gentle joint rotations can be done before exercise. Start from the toes and go all the way up to the neck. Do slow circular motions in clockwise and counter-clockwise until all the joints in the body can move smoothly. Bear in mind to keep everything in moderation and never take the rotations to the point where it can be painful.

Walk the Pain Away

Most health authorities list walking as the topmost form of exercise that can help ease the pain brought about by fibromyalgia. It is because walking is considered a low-impact exercise that is safe and easy to do. It improves blood circulation and can help bring oxygen to the muscles and decrease the stiffness as well as the pain.

Start by walking 10 minutes per day then gradually increase the duration to 30 minutes per day. It is best to walk every day at your most convenient time.

Warm Water Workout Can Be Good Too

Light exercise and warm water is a combination that can help soothe the pain away. According to research, women who do aquatic exercises in a heated pool for at least an hour thrice a week show fewer symptoms of fibromyalgia than those who did not do the workout.

Someone who would like to try the workout can start with ten minutes of warm up by walking in the water, followed by ten minutes of moderate water aerobics, twenty minutes of strength exercises then lastly, cooling down.

Stretch your Way to a Pain Free Life

Simple stretching, good posture and relaxation exercises can lessen the amount of pain. Take note that it is best to stretch the stiff muscles before and after completing a light aerobic exercise to avoid possible injury.

Stretch gently and make sure to never stretch to the point where it becomes painful. Hold the light stretches for 30 seconds. Daily stretching can provide a kind of lubrication to the joints and can send oxygen and nutrients to the muscles.

When stretching the calves, face the wall and place your hands flat against it (as if pushing the wall). Position your feet flat on the floor, with one foot in front of the other. Lean forward and feel the pull in your calves and Achilles tendons. Hold the position for thirty seconds and repeat the entire exercise two more times. Switch the position of the legs and repeat.

Lightly Lift

Strength training can also reduce the pain of fibromyalgia while improving the wellbeing of a person. Using resistance machines or lifting weights can benefit fibromyalgia patients a lot as long as the intensity is appropriate for the patient, it should be increased gradually and weights must be kept light.

Start at one to three pounds then slowly increase the weight and keep it under a manageable point; again, avoid overexertion.

Count in the Chores

If working out in a gym doesn't seem to give the expected benefits, then doing some chores in the house can also be considered as exercise for individuals with fibromyalgia. Activities like scrubbing and vacuuming can help ease the pain and improve bodily movement and function.

Doing at least thirty minutes of chores each day can help lessen the pain that fibromyalgia brings.

Isometrics

Sometimes regular strength training is painful, but an isometric chest press is another way to tone and strengthen your muscles. Isometric exercises involve tensing the muscles without stretching or moving the muscles.

Do the chest press by putting your arms at chest level then pressing your palms together as hard as you can. Hold the position for five seconds, and then take a five-second rest before repeating the whole cycle for at least four more times. Slowly build the time of holding the press up to 15 seconds (if not painful). Stop if the exercise brings in more pain.

There is no perfect exercise regimen for fibromyalgia patients. It is all a matter of trying many things out and finding what is best for you. When you discover the set of exercises that work for you, stick with it and make sure to do it regularly. For better guidance, you can also work with a physical therapist to come up with a personalized exercise routine.

Chapter 5 – Sugar: The Sweet Poison at the Root of It All

Glucose, fructose, sucrose, dextrose, lactose, brown rice syrup, corn syrup and cane juice: what do all of these have in common as well as 250 other chemical compounds? Sugar!! They are all examples of sugar - the sweet, delicious and natural substance commonly found in fruits, vegetables, dairy and grains. Sugar falls under the carbohydrate category of the food guide and is necessary in our body. Carbohydrates are the body's main source of energy which fuel all of our muscles and also our brain.

So how can something so delectable and natural be a problem? It might seem as though sugar is safe and good for the body since it comes from natural sources; but scientists have gathered proof that this sweet poison, contrary to popular belief, causes havoc in all of our cells when taken in excess. It is vital to look at the effects of sugar to the body in order to better understand how to conquer fibromyalgia.

According to Dr. Jacob Teitelbaum, MD from the Dr. Oz Show, an overgrowth of yeast or Candida is an underlying contributor to the incidence of fibromyalgia and other chronic conditions. Therefore, the solution is to rid the excessive growth of yeast from the body. However, just removing the excessive yeast is not enough because there will always be a certain amount left in the body. It is important to achieve a healthy balance of yeast in the digestive tract. To control the amount of yeast growth in the body, detoxing from sugar must be done since the primary food source of yeast is sugar.

The Problem with Too Much Sugar...

Sugar poses as a risk to our body and weakens our organs and immune system. It is estimated that sugar is around eight times more addictive than cocaine. It is a biological addiction, a disorder of the hormones and an error in the chemical balance in your body that causes cravings for sugars and other carbohydrates. Aside from the fact that sugar is the food source of yeast, sugar provides no nutritional benefits. Sugar is void of fiber, protein, minerals and enzymes. When you consume too much sugar, consequently, your body needs to make up for the lack of nutrients by borrowing these necessary nutrients, e.g. sodium, potassium, calcium and magnesium, from other parts of the body. You can imagine the long term effects on the body when it's trying to metabolize the constantly high amounts of sugar in it.

Probably the most dangerous thing about sugar is that it is in everything! Surprisingly, a can of tomato soup contains 4 teaspoons of sugar. You can find sugar hidden in peanut butter, tomato sauce, crackers, and many, many other products that would never seem to have a natural connection with sugar. Overconsumption fosters an acidic imbalance in our predominately alkaline body, which is another reason why sugar is a problem. I will go into further detail about alkalinity and acidity in the next chapter since understanding the pH balance in our body is crucial in order to combat fibromyalgia.

How Do You Know You're Addicted to Sugar?

A sugar addiction is connected with a persistent imbalance of blood sugar in the body. Below are observed behavioral and physiological symptoms of a sugar addiction:

- You have a craving for bread products, sugary beverages or sweets.

- You experience what is called a "food coma". It is the feeling of drowsiness and fatigue after a heavy meal when the body is trying to deal with the sugar influx.

- When you miss a meal, you get a feeling of lightheadedness. If your body is used to a high-energy, high-calorie intake during every meal, missing a meal can make your body go into withdrawal.

- After you eat something sweet, your body craves for more. This is due to the fructose in the sugar, which encourages the production of ghrelin, a substance that increases the feeling of hunger.

- You have become dependent on caffeine to get your body started. You keep looking for coffee and sodas in order to stay awake and keep going.

- You have a harder time losing weight compared to average people. This is not because of your genes and definitely not from being too fat. This is because your body is too busy dealing with all that sugar to actually start burning fat. Furthermore, the acidic environment created in your body makes it even harder to shed those pounds.

Usually, these can be alleviated or even completely removed by balancing your blood sugar. Here are the tried and tested methods to do just that:

- Eat more proteins. Protein promotes muscle-building and helps metabolize your excess fats.

- Eliminate sugar and empty carbohydrates from your diet. Eating healthy meals regularly should be sufficient for your energy needs.

- Eat more good fats, complex carbohydrates, fiber and essential nutrients. A craving for sugar can come from your body not getting enough nutrients. Fiber-rich foods are also great for detoxifying your body not only from the build-up of sugar, but also from fats and other toxins.

It is reported that sugar addiction is worse than other kinds of addiction. You might find that it is more difficult to win over your addiction since sugar is in almost everything you eat and drink. However, once you have decided to rid yourself of it, you'll see results that you will be proud of.

Now What??

There are a few options for treating the overgrowth of yeast and sugar in your body. A huge part of the equation is making a dietary lifestyle change. Some medical experts recommend Diflucan, an anti-fungal medication. You can consult your doctor about your condition and request for a prescription.

There are several books on Candida cleanses in the market that you can find. You could try " *Yeast Infection Guide: A Natural Candida Cure to Boost Your Immune System and Achieve Optimal Health with a Complete Candida Cleanse and Candida Diet*" by Lily Phillips.

Another absolute essential is having a sugar detox. For guidance, try the book " *21 Day Sugar Detox Guide for Beginners: Lose Weight Quickly, Achieve Optimal Health, Feel Energized and Eliminate Sugar Cravings Naturally*" by Emma Rose.

Consuming probiotics such as acidophilus will help maintain a healthy digestive environment. Acidophilus can be found in dairy products, particularly yogurt. Acidophilus supplements are also available at local pharmacies. Another exceptional product is consuming kefir, which is cow's milk fermented in specific bacteria resulting in a sour-tasting drink. This product can be found in health food stores.

Chapter 6 - Alkaline or Acidic?

In its basic sense, the alkaline diet (also known as the acid ash diet, alkaline ash diet and alkaline acid diet) is based on the theory that certain foods have a significant effect on the pH of our body fluids such as blood, saliva and urine.

When our body is in an alkaline state, it functions the way it was intended to. Almost all of the food products that we consume, once digested and metabolized, release either an alkaline base or an acid base into our blood. Grains, meat, shellfish, milk, poultry, cheese and salt all produce acid, hence unbalancing the proper pH of our blood (which is slightly alkaline). This kind of diet, if continued and not counteracted by alkaline foods, can cause some serious side effects.

There are at least 10 benefits to bringing your body into an alkaline state:

1. *Improves energy levels*

2. *Improves immune function*

3. *Slows aging*

4. *Reduces pain and inflammation*

5. *Decreases weight*

6. *Promotes teeth and gum health*

7. *Neutralizes acid imbalance*

8. *Eliminates risk factors for certain diseases*

9. *Improves overall heart condition*

10. *Removes harmful toxins*

After regulating their body's pH and eliminating foods that cause an influx of acid in the body, some people have reported a decrease in fibromyalgia symptoms. If the body's pH level falls below 7 or above 7.45, severe health conditions can occur with death being the worst outcome. When the pH falls below or above what is normal, the body constantly balances and fine tunes in order to keep this delicate balance. As a result, it will take nutrients from other areas of the body (such as the bones) and do whatever it needs to do to maintain its alkaline state. Consider it this way: when garbage is left out on the street, the rats come. In the same way, when our body is in an acidic state, our immunity is compromised. Wherever garbage is, diseases, cancers and abnormalities are sure to follow.

Let us take this information into consideration. The fastest way to heal fibromyalgia is to bring the body into an alkaline state. This is profound information and is not often talked about in media. Society has indeed a lot of learning to do. If you want to know more about the alkaline diet, you can try " *Alkaline Diet Guide: Lose Weight Quickly, Achieve Optimal Health and Feel Energized with the Alkaline Diet and Alkaline Recipes*" by Emma Rose.

Chapter 7 – The Power of Hydration

The natural healing power of hydration may not be a familiar natural treatment for fibromyalgia but it is by far more essential than any other treatment presented in this book. The topic of water is so foundational, so crucial, so revolutionary, that it deserves to have a chapter of its own. It is of utmost importance for people to be educated about the water they are consuming on a daily basis to nourish their bodies.

Our body's biology is composed of 75% water. Therefore, it is imperative to keep the body hydrated in order for all the cells, muscles and organs to function at their optimal levels. Surprisingly, not all water is created the same. Regardless of where you source your water, its basic chemical composition remains the same, H_2O. However, the structure of water is not created equal. Sometimes, your tap water may actually not be the best source water to consume. Globally, bottled watered is considered a popular alternative to tap water. In some countries, it is unsafe to consume the tap water because it is polluted with a variety of contaminants. When considering our water source, there are some important factors to consider such as its oxidation rating and its pH level.

First of all, it's important to note that plastic water bottles are one of the world's top pollutants. Only 1 out of 6 plastic bottles are actually recycled. This poses huge implications on the environment on many different levels. While this does not directly impact fibromyalgia, the long term repercussions can pose a lot of damage to our health and environment.

31

That being said, the plastic bottles that bottled water come in leech harmful chemicals into the contained water that contribute to raising estrogen levels in the human body. Due to the long process that involves production, packaging and transportation, the bottled water resides in its plastic bottle for lengthy periods of time. Therefore, the plastic chemicals have a longer window of time to leak into our water source. These are chemicals that should not be introduced into our body since they wreak havoc and create long term health implications.

Furthermore, bottled water and tap water in some areas have a higher positive oxidation rating which is correlated to an increase in free radicals in the body. These water sources are contributing to the problem of diseases and cancers rather than helping prevent them. It's horrifying to discover that the tap water in my city, which is considered top quality, is actually worse than the 7-Up soda in relation to its oxidation rating. 7-Up rated at least +400 while the tap water in my area rated over +600! Bottled water has almost the same oxidation rating as 7-Up and power drinks.

Besides the oxidation rating factor, it is also essential to take into account the pH level of the water we consume. The pH level in our water source is incredibly important, especially when we are looking at ways to heal fibromyalgia. Bottled water falls below neutral with 5/6 acidity. An acidic pH level is not good considering that our body is alkaline. Tap water's pH level will depend on where you live. In my area, where water is top quality, tap water is neutral at 7 on the pH scale. In some areas, the water is neutralized to reduce rusting of the water pipes (isn't that nice?).

In addition, chlorine is added to remove bacteria from the water since water poisoning is one of the top causes of death in the world. In the summer, the city increases the chlorine level to accommodate for the hotter climate. Consequently, the chlorine in the water is instantly absorbed into the body which may cause problems with our liver.

The beauty of alkaline water is that is supports the alkaline balance in our body. Unfortunately, only 1% of the world is educated about the positive, life changing effects of alkaline water. Achieving an alkaline state can quickly be achieved by drinking alkaline water. You can also partner alkaline water with a diet rich in alkaline foods – which should basically consist of food taken from plant sources like fruits and vegetables. Consuming alkaline water is greatly beneficial to our health. Its pH should be around 8.5-9.5. It hydrates the body more efficiently than bottled or tap water and it also detoxifies the body by neutralizing the acids and removing harmful toxins.

One of the best sources of alkaline water on the market right now is Kangen water. Kangen water uses a filter system that is attached to your sink in order to filter the water and create an alkaline pH level. In addition, the system ionizes the tap water through electrolysis which produces a negative oxidation rating. That means it becomes an antioxidant and takes away the harmful free radicals from the body. Furthermore, Kangen water can be used for cooking and cleaning. It's shocking to see all the pesticides and chemicals that wash off your vegetables after you use Kangen water to clean them.

When you get your hands on Kangen water, try a full body water transfusion. Drink 1 ounce for every pound of body weight a day. For an average 140 lb woman, that's about a gallon a day! Drink the same amount for 21 days and watch your body heal itself from the inside out. It's incredible!

Chapter 8 - Recommended Fibromyalgia Diet: Foods to Eat and to Avoid

Some foods can make fibromyalgia worse than before and there are also foods that can help ease the pain. Knowing which foods to avoid and to eat can bring great improvements on the symptoms of fibromyalgia.

Foods to Eat

Eating the right amounts of fruits, vegetables, fats, seeds, legumes, grains, lean meats, and fats can bring significant improvement in your overall health and fitness.

If you are committed to creating an alkaline environment in your body, consuming alkalizing foods will help you get there. Pretty much all fruits and vegetables are alkalizing – especially the green ones like wheat grass, kale, spinach, etc.

Try these excellent food choices:

- rich in fiber - green leafy vegetables, bran (particularly corn; also wheat, rice and oat), raw cauliflower, broccoli, cabbage, berries (particularly raspberries), celery, squash, beans (especially kidney beans), cooked white mushrooms, oranges, figs, nuts and seeds

- omega 3 – fish, soy beans, wheat germ, fortified milk, yogurt or eggs, beans, peas, tofu, nuts and seeds, canola oil, walnut oil and flaxseed oil

- lean protein – lean cuts of beef, lean ground beef, lean poultry (turkey, duck, chicken), lean pork and lean lamb

- antioxidants – black beans, pinto beans, berries, prunes, apples, pecans, sweet cherries, plums, cooked russet potatoes and artichokes

The trick is to keep everything balanced and avoid the foods that can worsen your fibromyalgial discomfort.

Foods to Avoid

Taking careful considerations on the foods to avoid can help a lot in alleviating the symptoms of fibromyalgia. Take note of the foods to eliminate in your diet and you will gain freedom from this debilitating condition.

Stop or minimize your consumption of sugar and artificial sweeteners. It's best to opt for stevia, a healthy and natural alternative for sugar without causing any trouble. You can also use natural sugar substitutes such as honey, agave syrup or even coconut sugar. Ultimately, sugar is a sweet poison to the body that causes inflammation and other diseases.

Drinks that contain caffeine must also go. Coffee, cola drinks and other caffeinated beverages should be avoided if you want to keep the pain away. If drinking coffee can't be avoided, choose the decaffeinated one. Keep in mind that caffeine can also be found in certain pain and cold medications so read their labels first before taking any of them.

Flavor enhancers like MSG and preservatives like sodium nitrate are bad news for people with fibromyalgia. To avoid foods that contain them, stay away from processed and canned foods and eat home-cooked meals instead when going to work or school.

It is also recommended to avoid milk-based products for a week if you have fibromyalgia. If you observe an improvement of your condition then you can do away with them. Get your daily dose of calcium from soy milk, tuna, broccoli, and salmon.

Eliminating gluten from the diet may also significantly improve the condition of some fibromyalgia patients. Anyone who would like to try a gluten-free diet should avoid pasta, grains, and white bread that contain wheat, barley or rye. These can be substituted with gluten-free alternatives such as corn or rice. Almond flour or coconut flour can also be used in baking instead of the usual wheat flour. Also, take note that some sauces may also contain gluten. Pay attention to ingredient labels. Wheat is surprisingly found in many products where you wouldn't think it would be.

Salt is also one thing that people with fibromyalgia should avoid. Experts know that bland food can make you lose interest in the whole endeavor therefore it is recommended to try eliminating salt in the diet gradually. Patients can also experiment with different salts, such as sea salt or Himalayan salt. Herbs and spices can also be used in creating unique flavors.

Monitor the foods that work best for you. It is best to keep a food journal and list down the foods that you have taken for the day and the events that happened on that particular day. Also, take special note of stress levels and the severity of the symptoms of your fibromyalgia.

Food Journal for Tracking Foods to Avoid

Creating a food journal is a great way to track your diet and changes in your symptom patterns. Include the following information in your food journal:

- Date
- Pain Scale (rate from 1 to 5 or 1 to 10)
- Details/Symptoms
- Food Eaten/# of Servings
- Triggers/Notes

Meal Guide

Sometimes it is difficult to plan for a healthy diet without a guide. The information below can help plan the right meal to take to ease the symptoms of fibromyalgia.

1. Fruit

Amount per Serving

-medium sized fresh fruit, one piece

-1/4 cup or 63 ml preserved or dried fruit

-1/2 cup (125 ml) fresh, frozen or canned fruit

Number of Servings

-ideally 4 or 5 per day

2. Greens

Amount per Serving

-1 cup raw green, leafy vegetables
-1/2 cup of cooked veggies, make sure not to overcook
-170 ml fruit or vegetable juice (preferably fresh)

Number of Servings
-ideally 4 or 5 per day

3. Grains

Amount per Serving
-a slice of bread (try spelt, buckwheat or corn bread)
-1 ounce dry cereal
-1/2 cup or 125 ml cooked cereal, pasta (try rice, corn or quinoa flour) or rice

Number of Servings
-ideally 6 to 8 per day

4. Fats

Amount per Serving

-1 tbsp (15ml) low-fat mayonnaise

-2 tbsp or 30 ml light salad dressing

-5 ml semi-melted margarine (that's about 1 tsp)

-1 tsp (5 ml) vegetable oil

Number of Servings
-ideally 2 to 3 per day

5. Seeds, including nuts and legumes

Amount per Serving

-1/3 cup (1.5 oz.) nuts (like almonds, pistachios, and peanuts)

-2 tbsp or 1/2 oz. sunflower seeds or other seeds

-1/2 cup cooked dry peas, beans or lentils

-2 tbsp or 30 ml peanut or almond butter

Number of Servings

-4 or 5 per week

6. Lean meat, poultry, fish or seafood

Amount per Serving

-1 ounce cooked lean meat, skinless poultry, fish or seafood

-1 egg

-1 ounce canned tuna in water without added salt

Number of Servings
-3 or less per day

Meal Plan

The meal plan below serves as your guide in planning your meal for the day (taken from the above meal guide).

Fruit (4-5 servings per day)

Breakfast: 170 ml fresh fruit juice

Snack (Optional): one fresh fruit

Lunch: ½ cup canned fruit

Snack (Optional): ¼ cup preserved fruit

Dinner: can add another serving here if desired

Greens (4-5 servings per day)

Breakfast: can have one serving here if desired

Snack (Optional): handful of cherry tomatoes

Lunch: 1/2 cup cooked mixed veggies

Snack (Optional): 170 ml fresh vegetable juice

Dinner: 1 cup raw green leafy vegetables

Grains (6-8 servings per day)

Breakfast: 3 slices of bread

Snack (Optional): 1 ounce dry cereal

Lunch: 1/2 cup steamed rice

Snack (Optional): 1 rice cake

Dinner: 1 cup cooked pasta

Fats (2-3 servings per day)

Breakfast: a tsp of semi-melted margarine

Dinner: olive oil salad dressing with a dash of lemon

Seeds including nuts and legumes (4-5 servings per week)

Breakfast: sprinkle flax seeds or chia seeds on your cereal or a smoothie; spread almond or peanut butter on your toast

Snack (Optional): almonds or pumpkin seeds

Snack (Optional): peanut butter or almond butter

Lean meat (2-3 servings per day)

Breakfast: 1 poached egg

Lunch: 2 ounces fish

Snack (Optional): 1 hard boiled or scrambled egg

Dinner: 2 ounces lean meat

Ways to Enjoy Your Meat

The best way to cook your lean meat is by grilling, steaming or broiling. Avoid frying them as much as possible and if you need to add some sugar or salt, keep it minimal.

For fish, it can be steamed and served with a light mayo dip to enjoy a succulent dish.

For added taste, you can also prepare a dry rub for the meat – a bit of salt, chili powder and pepper. Spread the dry rub all over the meat then grill or broil it. Prepare a light salad to complete your meal. The dry rub goes well with any meat including fish.

Create some variations in taste by squeezing a lemon or lime on the meat before cooking.

As you go along with the planning and preparing of the healthy dishes to keep the symptoms of fibromyalgia under control, you will see that everything will become natural and easier to you.

Following a healthy meal plan will not only improve the symptoms of fibromyalgia but the overall fitness and health as well (not to mention the bonus of having a slim and fit body).

It is said that it takes 21 days to break a habit. Try maintaining your dietary changes for at least 21 days to see results. Expect to have symptoms of withdrawal if you choose to cut out caffeine, sugar, dairy or wheat. Sometimes you may feel worse before you actually feel better. Stick with it because it will soon pass and the reward will be worth it.

Chapter 9 - Recipes to Try

Gone are the days when eating healthy and nutritious food is synonymous with something bland and unappetizing. With some help from these great healthy recipes and good meal planning, putting an end to the hardships brought about by fibromyalgia will just take a fraction of time.

Here are some recipes to try and include in your meal plan. You can divide the prepared food to eat during lunch and dinner, just make sure not to go way beyond the suggested serving portions.

Berry Salad and Blackened Chicken

You will need:

2 ounces of skinless chicken breast

1/2 tsp mixture of blackening spice

½ head romaine lettuce

Vegetable toppings (radish, grated carrots, tomato, peas, pea pods, red cabbage and pepper strips)

fruit toppings (raspberries, blueberries and strawberry slices)

olive oil

vinegar or lemon dressing

Procedure:

Get the chicken breast and rub it with the blackening spice mixture. Grill until internal temperature has reached 165°F.

Prepare the salad base using the romaine lettuce. Top with the vegetable toppings, then the fruit toppings. Add oil and vinegar dressing or olive oil with lemon dressing. This is good for a single serving.

Tuna Salad Platter

You will need:

1 ounce canned tuna in water

1/4 cup celery, chopped

2 tbsp light mayonnaise (or yogurt for a healthier choice)

1 hard boiled egg

bell pepper strips, shredded cabbage, cherry tomatoes, grated carrots

1 cup romaine lettuce, divided in two parts

Procedure:

Mix tuna, celery, mayonnaise and egg then set aside. Toss half of the romaine lettuce at the bottom of a salad bowl and top with half of the sliced vegetables. Toss in the other half of the romaine and then half of the sliced vegetables. Add in the previously prepared tuna and mayonnaise dressing.

Tuna Salad with Jalapeño

You will need:

1 6-ounce canned tuna in water, drained

1 tbsp light mayonnaise (or yogurt for a healthier choice)

1 small jalapeño, diced and without seeds

1 small tomato, diced

1/2 tbsp lime juice

1/4 onion, finely chopped

Procedure:

Put tuna in a bowl then add mayonnaise and onion. Mix them well. Add the remaining ingredients and serve.

Grilled Crunchy Chicken

You will need:

2 ounces chicken breast, with the skin on

A clove of garlic

Seasoning mix without salt

Aluminum foil

Procedure:

Rub the chicken breast with garlic and the salt-free seasoning. Heat the grill using medium heat. Make a "boat" for the breast using the aluminum foil. Put the chicken in the boat and place the aluminum boat on the grill. Cook for 45 minutes while turning the chicken inside the boat every fifteen minutes. When chicken turns golden brown, serve.

This makes 2 servings.

Stuffed Colorful Peppers

You will need:

3 pcs bell pepper (red, green, and yellow)

350 grams lean ground beef or sirloin

1 egg

2 tablespoons oat bran

1-2 cloves garlic, crushed

1 tsp paprika

Procedure:

Preheat your oven to 356ºF or 180ºC. While preheating your oven, cut your bell peppers in half, lengthwise. Deseed the bell peppers. Line your roasting tin with wax paper or greaseproof paper. Arrange your sliced bell peppers on the tin. Bake them for approximately 10-15 minutes. While baking your bell peppers, prepare the beef stuffing. In your food processor, place your beef, egg, oat bran, paprika and garlic. Mix these ingredients well. In the absence of a food processor, you may also mix the ingredients in a bowl. Use a fork to mix well. Take out the bell peppers from the oven and let them cool a bit. Stuff them with the beef mixture and put them back in the oven. Bake for approximately 20-30 minutes or until the beef mixture is done.

Mushroom Burger

You will need:

8 oz. of lean ground beef or sirloin

6-8 pcs Portobello mushroom

2 tablespoons oat bran

2 strips low fat bacon

1 tablespoon flaxseed

1 teaspoon olive oil

Procedure:

In a bowl, mix all ingredients well except the mushroom and bacon. Form patties out of the mixture. Grill your patties and bacon. Remove the stems of your mushrooms. Arrange your stemless mushrooms on a pan neatly. Set your stove on medium-high and cook your mushroom until the juices come out. Place one burger patty on two mushrooms. Add the bacon on top of the patty then top it with another mushroom.

Egg and Spinach Scramble

You will need:

1-2 eggs, beaten

½ cup baby spinach, chopped

¼ teaspoon cumin

1 small clove of garlic, minced

½ medium-sized white onion

½ tablespoon dried onion

1 teaspoon virgin coconut oil

Procedure:

Mix the eggs, baby spinach, cumin and dried onion in a bowl. In a heated pan, put your virgin coconut oil and sauté garlic and onion. Add the egg mixture. Cook for 2-3 minutes.

Primal Breakfast Burrito

You will need:

4 egg whites

1 to 2 tomatoes, finely chopped

½ medium-sized onion, finely chopped

1 red pepper, cut into strips

¼ cup canned and diced green chilies

½ a cup of cooked meat (you can use ground beef, sliced steak or shredded chicken)

¼ cup of chopped cilantro

hot sauce or salsa

1 avocado cut into wedges

Procedure:

First, whisk your egg whites. Then, lightly oil a 10-inch skillet and warm this over a low fire. Slowly pour half of your egg whites onto the pan, making sure to swirl it so that it gets spread evenly and thinly. Cook it for about a minute until it resembles a tortilla before removing it from the pan. This would be your burrito wrapper. Using the same pan, sauté your onions in oil before adding the red pepper, tomato, green chili and meat. Whisk more of the egg yolks into this and turn it into a scramble along with your other ingredients. Spoon half of this filling into your wrapper and roll it up nice and tight. Add some avocados on top and serve with salsa or hot sauce.

Veggies with Spinach Artichoke Dip

You will need:

10 ounces frozen and chopped spinach

2 14-ounce cans of artichoke hearts

half a red bell pepper

1 teaspoon garlic powder

1/2 cup cashew butter

1 tablespoon of green onion

¼ teaspoon cayenne

1 teaspoon salt

Procedure:

Cook your frozen spinach over medium heat, slowly breaking it up while it cooks. Add your red bell and artichokes and mix until everything is heated through. Then, add in your butter, cashew, garlic, cayenne, salt and green onion. Stir thoroughly and evenly. Serve this with your choice of veggies or veggie chips.

Sesame Seed Crusted Snapper

You will need:

6 to 7 ounces Red snapper, filleted and skinned

1 tablespoon sesame seeds

kosher or sea salt,

fresh black pepper (cracked)

1 tablespoon of grass-fed butter

Procedure:

Dust one side of the snapper fillet with a mixture of kosher salt and pepper before laying it on top of the sesame seeds. Press down to ensure an even coating. Do the same to the other side. In a frying pan, melt a teaspoon of the butter. Increase the heat before putting the snapper in the pan, cooking each side for at least 3 to 4 minutes. The seeds should take on a golden color.

Honey Orange Chicken

Ingredients:

1 pound chicken breast, cubed

2 tablespoons garlic

2 tablespoons ginger

2 tablespoons honey

2 tablespoons coconut aminos

1 tablespoon chili sauce

1/2 cup orange juice

green onions, chopped

fish sauce for seasoning

How to:

Stir fry your chicken in the coconut oil until it begins to brown. Add your garlic and ginger then sauté for 1 minute. Lower your heat and add the liquid ingredients. Stir everything to coat the chicken evenly and allow to simmer until the sauce thickens. Serve with green onions.

Spinach and Ham Omelet with Spicy Piperade

You will need:

coconut oil

2 eggs already beaten

salt and pepper

1 cup ham, cubed

at least a handful of baby spinach torn into small pieces

Procedure (Omelet):

Melt your coconut oil using a small sauté pan then add your eggs. Season the eggs with some salt and pepper. Cook it until your egg has set then sprinkle it with ham and pile on the spinach to one side. After you've placed the ham and spinach on one side, fold the egg. Top this with piperade.

You will need (Piperade):

3 cloves garlic

a large onion

3 tablespoons olive oil

4 sprigs of thyme

1 red bell pepper

1 yellow bell pepper

1 red chilli

1 cup cherry tomatoes

1 teaspoon salt

Procedure (Piperade):

Sauté your garlic, onions and thyme in the olive oil and wait until your onion begins to soften. After, add your chilli and peppers, continue to sauté this for at least 3 more minutes before finally adding the tomatoes. Sprinkle some salt to taste before covering and letting it simmer for at least 5 minutes.

Mango Avocado Spiced Chicken Salad

You will need:

1 small lettuce

1 to 2 cups of shredded chicken

1 diced avocado

1 diced mango

½ teaspoon cumin

½ teaspoon chili powder

salt and pepper for seasoning

Procedure:

Place your lettuce in a bowl and do the same to your chicken in a separate one. Add a tiny bit of water to your chicken to keep it moist before microwaving for at least 15 seconds. Add the chili and cumin to this and mix. Once done, add it to your lettuce and simply top with some avocadoes and mangoes. You can add a light dressing such as olive oil and lemon juice, or eat as is.

Conclusion

Thank you again for purchasing *"Fibromyalgia Book Guide."*

I hope this book was able to help you find treatments and strategies on how to successfully live with fibromyalgia and manage your pain.

The next step is to apply these strategies and make the necessary changes to your diet. It's shocking how the food we eat has such profound effects on the body -especially sugar. I'm amazed by how much better my body feels after cutting sugar out of my diet even for just 2 weeks. Although it was incredibly difficult for me to do, I came to a point of desperation which propelled me to make the changes necessary for my health.

Finally, if you enjoyed this book and found it meaningful, please take the time to share your thoughts and post a positive review on Amazon. I greatly appreciate your time and effort. If you want free books and want to know what some of my friends and I are up to, please like our Facebook page: www.facebook.com/joypublishing

I would love for you to share your experiences, stories and encouragements with me. My email address is miasoleilkindle@gmail.com

In addition, please remember to check out our Facebook page in order to find other resources and upcoming promotions:

https://www.facebook.com/joypublishing

Sincerely,

Mia Soleil

Preview Of "Eczema Treatment Guide"

Chapter 1 – What is Eczema?

Eczema is frequently confused with another skin condition known as psoriasis, but the two are simply not the same. To differentiate them, the adult eczema is usually found on the flexor portion of the joints in the body or those parts on the inner side of a joint that can reduce in size or area due to flexing. Alternatively, psoriasis is not commonly found in those parts.

Eczema is a kind of dermatitis which refers to the inflammation of the outermost layer of the skin or the epidermis. It is a condition in which certain portions of the skin become irritated and scabrous. The skin can break out in blisters that cause itchiness and bleeding. This may be due to the skin's reaction to an irritant medically referred to as eczematous dermatitis. However, more commonly the condition may emerge without evident environmental or external cause.

This skin problem usually begins during the early years but it can also start later in life. Eczema is typically identified with dry, severely itchy, red-colored patches on the skin. Because some people, especially the young kids, cannot avoid scratching when the patches of skin become itchy, they tend to have rashes.

Chapter 2 - Causes of Eczema

There must be some sort of trigger that brings about the eruption of the irritating red-colored lesions commonly observed among people who are suffering from eczema. For instance, a break out of contact dermatitis may have been caused by something as outwardly safe as being dressed in garments made of coarse fabric. These rough clothing may be made of wool or other materials like it. Moreover, cigarettes or tobacco, soaps with strong chemicals, bleach, smoke, animal fur or hair, and other chemical substances can trigger the break out of eczema. This can particularly occur among little children who are vulnerable to this type of skin condition.

The major causes of majority of the usual types of eczema are hereditary in nature. One parent or both of them may have experienced this skin problem due to allergic reactions like runny nose and asthmatic attacks. This kind of susceptibility can be passed on from one generation to the next.

Even if eczema is usually a hereditary condition, a flare-up is also contingent to the type of condition a patient has.

Atopic eczema or infantile eczema – This is the most prevalent form that is known to be hereditary. It is usually seen among kids whose immune system may be severely reacting to certain triggers like flakes of the skin, animal hair or fur, dust mites, pollen, among others. Exposure can result to inflamed, chafed, and itchy skin.

Contact dermatitis – This is brought about by contact with any irritant which can set off skin eruptions.

Xerotic eczema – This is not a common type and affects the elderly. It is caused by skin dryness that usually occurs at a certain season of the year. The skin becomes dry and ultimately breaks out.

Other types

Neurodermatitis – This type manifests with inflamed red-colored lichen eczema typically caused by continuous scratch and rub actions.

Dyhidrosis - This type of eczema is concentrated on the palms, the sides of the fingers, and the soles of the feet. It feels itchier during the night.

Venous eczema – This commonly occurs among individuals aged above fifty years old whose circulation is impeded.

Discoid eczema – This condition aggravates during extreme cold weather and is characterized by lesions on the lower portion of the leg.

Determining the Cause

Allergy testing under medical supervision is a wide-ranging method that can precisely isolate the cause of an eczema problem. Aside from determining one's allergies, this kind of test will also determine the personal reactions of a particular individual to certain allergens like molds, pollens, or drugs. This test will be able to indicate what it is you are exactly allergic to. This might take some time before results are obtained. The medical practitioner working on you might have found numerous allergens which you might be reacting to; hence, the process may not be completed as fast as you want it to.

Taking this test is not only beneficial for exactly determining the kinds of food products or substance in them that you are reacting against. This will also determine any factor in the environment that may also be triggering your eczema. Among these environmental factors are smoke, dust mites, pollen, and some chemicals found in hygiene and cleaning products.

Naturopaths have been known to request blood work for their patients in order to determine whether there are specific foods that are triggering the eczema.

Check out the rest of this book on Amazon.

Or go to: http://www.amazon.com/Eczema-Treatment-Guide-Natural-Treatments-ebook/dp/B00J46JSOK

PAIN MANAGEMENT

How to Achieve Pain Relief & Live Pain Free for Life

MIA SOLEIL

© **Copyright 2014 by Joy Publishing & Marketing Corporation - All rights reserved.**

This document is geared towards providing helpful and reliable information in regards to the topic and issue covered. The publication is sold with the idea that the publisher is not required to render accounting, officially permitted, or otherwise, qualified services. If advice is necessary, legal or professional, a practiced individual in the profession should be ordered.

- From a Declaration of Principles which was accepted and approved equally by a Committee of the American Bar Association and a Committee of Publishers and Associations.

In no way is it legal to reproduce, duplicate, or transmit any part of this document in either electronic means or in printed format. Recording of this publication is strictly prohibited and any storage of this document is not allowed unless with written permission from the publisher. All rights reserved.

The information provided herein is stated to be truthful and consistent, in that any liability, in terms of inattention or otherwise, by any usage or abuse of any policies, processes, or directions contained within is the solitary and utter responsibility of the recipient reader. Under no circumstances will any legal responsibility or blame be held against the publisher for any reparation, damages, or monetary loss due to the information herein, either directly or indirectly.

Respective authors own all copyrights not held by the publisher.

The information herein is offered for informational purposes solely, and is universal as so. The presentation of the information is without contract or any type of guarantee assurance.

The trademarks that are used are without any consent, and the publication of the trademark is without permission or backing by the trademark owner. All trademarks and brands within this book are for clarifying purposes only and are the owned by the owners themselves, not affiliated with this document

Table of Contents

Introduction — 1

Pain and the Body — 3

Pain Management in Medical Context — 7

How Does Pain Affect your Life? — 9

Natural Pain Relievers — 11

What Aggravates Pain? — 17

How to Prevent Relapses — 21

Understanding TMS — 23

Conclusion — 43

One Last Thing... — 45

Introduction

I want to thank you and congratulate you for purchasing the book, "**PAIN MANAGEMENT**: How to Achieve Pain Relief & Live Pain Free for Life".

This book contains proven steps and strategies on how to recognize and differentiate types of pain and their causes. The main insight this book will provide, the one that we're all craving for, is how to achieve pain relief. The goal was to create a book rich in practical techniques and strategies for achieving the relief from pain that we all so desperately desire. Once we are able to bring our bodies into a pain free reality, the challenge is to prevent relapse. We'll conclude with strategies for promoting this lasting change.

I personally have struggled with chronic pain in the forms of lower back and neck pain, and headaches. From Elementary to Secondary school, I had a headache almost every day. I actually didn't know what it was like to NOT have a headache. I frequently took pain relieving medicines like Tylenol and Advil to help cope with the daily pain. In the end, it was actually my sinuses that were contributing to the problem all along. Once I was able to deal with the root of the problem, rather than the symptoms, I saw a drastic turn around.

I also had a serious accident that was so powerful, I knocked down a lamp post! I didn't feel the effects of this car accident till about six years later. The accident and progression of poor posture and stress caused my chronic neck pain to rear its ugly head. That led to a sloughs of chiropractor and massage therapy appointments over the next several years.

In December 2010, I gave birth to my daughter. I was originally very scared of the anticipated pain of childbirth. I couldn't imagine how it would all physically take place. Through a series of events and an adjustment of my thinking, which I'll save for another book, I was able to be at peace with labor. I successfully gave birth naturally, in my own home, without any form of pain medication. Keep in mind: this is coming from the same person that would take Tylenol for a simple headache because I was such a wimp when it came to dealing with pain.

Our lives should not be crippled because of pain. We shouldn't have to settle for less than awesome because of the debilitating effects of chronic pain in our daily lives. We shouldn't have to sit on the sidelines because we're in too much pain to play the game. Everyone that has been on this journey knows the cost of trying to achieve a pain free life – it is a costly one. It stops here! My hope for you is that this is the last price to be paid on your chronic pain.

I sincerely thank you for purchasing this book. I truly hope you enjoy it! I hope you are able to gain insight, encouragement and strategies to apply to your life to receive the joy and peace you deserve.

Please take some time to stop by and LIKE our Facebook page:

https://www.facebook.com/joypublishing

With gratitude,

Mia Soleil

Chapter 1

Pain and the Body

When you cut yourself, blood oozes out and there's a sharp pain that follows. If you have a migraine, you feel a chronic throbbing pain in your head. If you are burnt, pain is intensely unbearable. These are different scenarios where a person undergoes a painful experience. Pain in varying degrees of intensity and frequency is identified. The definition of pain, however, is out of the question.

What is Pain?

Pain is a complex stimulus. There is no exact definition because it is an entirely subjective sensation. It is the foremost reason why people seek medical attention. Pain tells you that something is wrong or damaged. The International Association for the Study of Pain defines it as "an unpleasant sensory and emotional experience associated with actual or potential tissue damage or described in terms of such damage".

In actual context, pain is not always associated with physiological processes. Medical attention can identify and treat physical pain, but there's also another kind of pain which is really hard if not impossible to treat through medical means...emotional pain. So what is pain? Pain, to put it simply, is far more than neural transmission and sensory transduction. It is a complex mixture of emotion, sensation, culture, experience and spirit.

How Does the Body React to Pain?

Pain perception or nociception is the process where a painful stimulus is signaled and relayed to the central nervous system from the point of origin. It is entirely different when compared to normal stimuli like touch, ordinary pressure and temperature.

When the stimulus is non-painful, normal somatic receptors are the first to act. If it is a painful stimulation, nociceptors are the first to fire up.

This process includes several steps:

1. *Point of origin or contact with stimulus* - the point of origin can be mechanical such as cuts, pressures, abrasions and pressure. It can also be chemically inflicted like burns.

2. *Reception* - It is a process where the nerve ending senses the stimulus.

3. *Transmission* - When nerve endings sense the stimulus, they transmit the signal to the central nervous system through a series of neurons.

4. *Perception* - This is where the brain receives the signal for further processing and action.

When you cut your hand, there are several factors that contribute to your perception of pain. First is the mechanical stimulation of the sharp object that cut you. Your cells are damaged and they release potassium. This is why you feel the intense sharp pain at the moment of injury. Then Prostaglandins, histamines and bradykinins from the immune cells invade the area during inflammation. This is the stage where your body is protecting you from the foreign stimulus. You will experience a longer dull ache or numbing feeling along the affected area.

Nociceptor neurons travel in peripheral sensory nerves. The signals are relayed from the free nerve endings at the layer of the skin. These signals are sent to the spinal cord through the dorsal roots. They synapse on the neurons within the spinal cord segment and also two or three segments below and above the point of entry. This is basically the reason why it is sometimes difficult to locate the location of the pain in the body especially when the damage is internal.

Secondary neurons then transmit the signal upward through the spinothalamic tract. The signal travels from the spinothalamic tract to the medulla (brain's system) and ends in the thalamus, which is the central relaying center of the brain. Some neurons also send signal to the medulla's reticular receptors which control the physical behavior.

Once the signal is processed in the brain, some signals will pass through the motor cortex, to the spinal cord then down to the motor nerves. These impulses cause muscle contractions that make you move your hand away from the object.

What are the Types of Pain?

There are different types of pain. Neuroscientists and physicians classify pain in three ways:

1. *Acute Pain* - This is a type of pain which is inflicted to the body. An injury to the body like a cut or burn causes an acute pain in the affected area. It warns of potential damage and compels action from the brain. It can develop slowly or quickly. Depending on the type of injury and the intensity of the damage, pain can last up to a few minutes to a year. When the wound starts to heal however, acute pain goes away.

2. *Chronic Pain* - It is a persistent kind of pain. It does not require your body to respond unlike acute pain. Chronic pain still persists even when the trauma has been healed. It lasts longer than six months. An example of a chronic pain is a migraine.

3. *Cancer/Malignant Pain* - This is a kind of pain associated with tumors. It is somehow associated with chronic pain; however, cancer pain is more painful and affects a wider area. This is because tumors invade healthy cells thus, affecting nearby blood vessels and nerves.

Chapter 2

Pain Management in Medical Context

When a person goes to a hospital for pain treatment, physicians treat it in numerous possible ways. Pain management consists of medication such as taking an aspirin or ibuprofen as a pain reliever; surgery, which is common to more serious injuries like gunshots, burns, and organ failures; alternative procedures like hypnosis, massage therapy and acupuncture; or a combination of these approaches.

The type of medication prescribed depends on the source of pain, side effects of the medication, health status of the person and the level of discomfort experienced by the afflicted.

1. **Medication**: There are different types of medication given to a patient at a certain time and scenario.

   - *Non-Opioid Analgesics* - This includes aspirin, ibuprofen, acetaminophen and naproxen. They are used as pain relievers and they act on the site of pain directly. When the tissue is damaged, an enzyme is released and local pain or the pain on the affected area is produced. This type of medication prevents the onset of these enzymes, soothes the pain and reduces inflammation. This type of analgesics, however, can have adverse effects on the kidneys and liver and causes internal bleeding and gastrointestinal discomfort when usage is prolonged.

- *Opioid Analgesics* - This medication is applied to higher and more intense levels of pain. They act on the synaptic neurons and activate downward pathways of signals. They target various parts in the central nervous system by binding to Opioid receptors. This includes morphine, codeine, meripidine, fentanyl, propoxyphine, and oxycodone. The side effect can be addictive and over dosage is likely to occur at different times.

- *Adjuvant Analgesics* - These are also pain relievers but they are used to treat other conditions. They act against neuropathic pain or the pain caused by damage to the central nervous system. This includes tricyclic anti-depressants, anti-epileptic drugs and anesthetics.

2. **Surgery**: Surgery is always the last resort. When all the pain relievers no longer alleviate pain, surgery must be done to sever pain pathways. Two types of surgery include Rhizotomy, which destroys portions of the peripheral nerves; and Achordotomy, which destroys ascending tracts to the spinal cord preventing the pain signal receptors in reaching the medulla or the brain system.

3. **Alternative Therapy**: This does not involve drugs or surgery. It includes chiropracty (manipulates joints to relieve nerve pressures), massage, hot compress, acupuncture (stimulates nerves and release endorphins) and mental control such as hypnosis which rely on the brain to alleviate pain.

Chapter 3

How does pain affect your Life?

Pain can affect your life in numerous ways. If you are a professional and have to go to work, if you experience pain, your work is affected. You will not be able to concentrate on finishing your tasks if something is wrong with you. If you are sick, you have to be absent for treatment or rest. Either way, your work is still affected. If you are a parent, how can you take care of your kids if you are hurt? Pain, is of course a natural stimulus that should not be taken for granted. The more you ignore the pain, the worse your situation may become.

If pain is chronic, it has a detrimental effect on the everyday life of the person. It affects the patient's ability to perform natural functions and responsibilities. Physical activities are limited. Chronic pain is also associated with depression, anxiety, sleep disturbances and panic attacks. Chronic pain also impedes mobility or flexibility of the patient as it may result to difficulty in walking or carrying things, poor personal hygiene, and loss of social contacts with family and friends, and constipation and incontinence.

Chronic pain affects you physically and psychologically. It limits what you can do. It interferes with your ability to work, play with your children or grandchildren; it also diminishes your ability to take care of your own self. When these happen, pain causes you to feel useless and incompetent, making you succumb to a depressed state. People with chronic pain often experience irritability, anger, depression, and difficulty in concentrating. It becomes as debilitating as the pain itself.

Pain changes a person's personality. Coping with chronic pain, on the other hand, calls for a great deal of change and introspection from the person itself. It pressures the person while he is trying to hide the pain and forces himself to cover the handicap by a sense of forged well-being to be functional.

- The Pain Haze - Chronic pain is unpredictable. It is sometimes mild and other times, it is unbearable. When a person is in pain, his perception about things is obscured and his responses are slow. This is the stage where a person's personality does not reflect on the outside.

- Mental Health Condition - Pain causes sleeplessness and mood swings. Chronic pain leads to painful depressions and helplessness which, in turn leads to suicidal tendencies, anxiety and panic disorders.

- Perception - People who are in painful situations are always misunderstood. Oftentimes, their real perception and intentions are not reflected on the outside. Their ways of coping with pain is essentially vital to how people view them. Their view of life is also affected. Those who suffer from serious illnesses perceive life as something they have to live to the fullest as their time is already counted and the likes. Some also become hopeless and afraid of the things to come.

Chapter 4

Natural Pain Relievers

There are many circumstances where prescribed medications just won't work. There are also times when your body does not respond positively to treatments. If you have allergic reactions to certain medications, especially pain relievers and anesthetics, it is best that you use natural alternatives instead for pain treatment. Nature is still the best healer. There are wonderful herbs out there that contain extracts effective in reducing inflammation and infection. Here are a few of them:

1. *Capsaicin*: This is an active component found in chili pepper. It temporarily desensitizes C fibers which are the pain-prone nerve receptors. If applied on the injured area, Capsaicin diminishes soreness for three to five weeks until the nerves regain sensation. It has already been proven effective and is now commercially sold and used worldwide. It has been reported that forty percent of arthritis patients experienced fifty percent pain reduction after one month of using capsaicin cream.

2. *Inflathera and Zyflamend*: These two components are both present in ginger, turmeric and holy basil which are all anti-inflammatory agents. Turmeric, which is also an ingredient used primarily in delicious curry meals, is one of the best natural pain relievers. New research suggests that turmeric contains curcumin, which eases inflammatory conditions like rheumatoid arthritis and psoriasis. It also has anti-cancer properties. Furthermore, turmeric also helps in blood circulation and prevents blood clotting. Curcumin lowers the amount of enzymes released by the damaged cells and reduces the pain in the body. It is best used to treat, bruises, joint inflammation, skin and digestive issues. Ginger on the other hand, has been used

to relieve pain since thousands of years ago by the Chinese people. It relieves nausea, arthritis, headaches, menstrual cramps, muscle soreness and blood circulation issues.

3. *Valerian Root*: Valerian root is also called nature's tranquilizers. It regulates the central nervous system thereby relieving insomnia, tension, irritability or mood swings, anxiety and stress. A cup of Valerian aids in pain relief by reducing sensitivity of the nerves.

4. *Salicin*: This is a component commonly found in aspirins. It is also naturally found in white willow barks. This traditional pain reliever is used to treat painful joint inflammation. White willow bark effects are slower than the commercial aspirin but it is much longer. Contrary to aspirin, white willow bark does not upset the stomach and won't damage gastro-intestinal lining. It was also discovered that white willow bark reduces the severity of migraine attacks.

5. *Arnica*: Arnica is a component found active in a European flower. Although the healing mechanism remains unknown, it does contain anti-inflammatory properties. This is best applied to relieve acute injury or post-surgery swelling. Taking oral homeopathic arnica after a surgery reduces painful swelling.

6. *Herbal and Fish Oil*: Herbal or Tonic oil such as peppermint, camphor, eucalyptus, fennel and wintergreen can be used to treat migraine or normal headaches. They can be applied topically on the affected area and their menthol or cooling properties reduce pain and inflammation. Digested fish oils on the other hand, when broken down, become prostaglandin, which are powerful agents that reduce inflammation. In one study, about 40 percent of patients suffering from rheumatic arthritis who have taken cod-liver oil for a month were able to cut their

NSAIDS intake by a third. Two-thirds of people who experience neck and back pains were able to stop using NSAIDS altogether after 10 weeks of taking cod-liver fish oil.

7. *Methysulfonyl-Methane (MSM)*: This is an active component of sulfur and it prevents joint and cartilage degeneration. In an experiment conducted by the University of California in San Diego, scientists reported that people with osteoarthritis who took MSM have experienced twenty-five percent less pain and are thirty percent more physically active than their counterparts who didn't.

8. *Apple Cider Vinegar*: This contains alkaline forming properties necessary for the body. One tablespoon of apple cider vinegar relieves the person of the painful spasms caused by heart burn. It also contains over-all alkalizing effects which the body desperately needs during this modern era of acid-forming diets.

9. *Bromelain*: An active component of pineapple, it is known to relieve bloated tummy and heaviness. It also improves blood circulation, preventing blood clots, inhibits inflammation, and stops muscle and menstrual cramps. It is recommended to those who suffer from arthritis.

10. *Garlic*: In the olden times, garlic was the most popular pain reliever. It is a home remedy for tooth-ache and other skin problems such as psoriasis and acne. Garlic contains anti-fungal and anti-inflammatory properties that are best for pain treatment and healing.

11. *Oats*: Oats are believed to have powerful effects in the reduction of menstrual cramps. It also relives endometriosis. They contain magnesium and are the best

sources of dietary zinc necessary for women who always suffer from painful menstrual periods.

12. *Grapes*: An Ohio University research study shows that 1 cup of grapes when eaten on a daily basis reduces the risks and frequency of suffering from back pains. They are said to contain nutrients that aid in the blood circulation, thus alleviating pain.

13. *Blueberries*: They contain anti-oxidants which kill free radicals that enflame the digestive lining, thereby reducing severity of gastrointestinal pain.

In addition to this long list of natural pain relievers, are several practitioners that you may already familiar with. Some of these services complement each other. Often chronic pain is a compounded and complex issue. It's like an onion with several layers. It is not uncommon to partner several of these services together. They all support each other in helping peel away the layers.

1. *Chiropracty*: Chiropractors focus on the neuromusculoskeletal system and the connection the spine has with the rest of the body. They believe that misalignment or subluxations can even occur during the process of birth. When our body is out of alignment, chronic conditions and pain is created in the body. The chiropractor physically manipulates the joints to relieve nerve pressure and facilitate healing. Often, the muscles around the spine need to be taught to have a "new memory" so that pain relief can be maintained.

2. *Massage Therapy*: massage therapy can often go hand in hand with other forms of physical therapy. The practice focuses on manipulating the muscles and connective tissues in the body through a variety of techniques. The American Heritage dictionary says "massage is the rubbing

or kneading of parts of the body to aid circulation or relax the muscles." Chronic pain can be alleviated when the muscles are relaxed and able to function as they were designed. Massage therapy can come in many forms such as deep tissue massage, Swedish massage, Shiatsu and many more.

3. *Chinese Medicine*: Chinese medicine is based on 5000 years of tradition. It usually encompasses herbal medicine, acupuncture, massage, exercise and diet.

4. *Acupuncture/Acupressure*: stimulates nerves and release endorphins based on the different pressure points in the body. Acupuncture places needles into the skin along specific meridians and acupuncture points. Acupressure uses fingers, hands or other instruments instead of needles.

5. *Physiotherapy*: it is not uncommon to use physiotherapy after some form of serious accident that has disabled the body in some way. Usually after an accident, the body has a limited range of motion or is not able to perform the way it was intended. Physiotherapy treats the body's disease, injury or deformity by the means of physical techniques rather than drugs or surgery. These techniques include massage, stretching, exercise and heat treatment.

6. *Naturopathy*: According to the Canadian Association of Naturopathic Doctors, "naturopathic medicine is a distinct primary health care system that blends modern scientific knowledge with traditional and natural forms of medicine. The naturopathic philosophy is to stimulate the healing power of the body and treat the underlying cause of disease. Symptoms of disease are seen as warning signals of improper functioning of the body, and unfavorable lifestyle habits. In addition to diet and lifestyle changes, natural therapies including botanical medicine, clinical

nutrition, hydrotherapy, homeopathy, naturopathic manipulation and traditional Chinese medicine or acupuncture, may also be used during treatments."

7. *Aromatherapy*: there is a powerful connection between the olfactory system and the aroma of essential oils. Different herbs have different healing properties that are capable of treating a variety of chronic conditions. Aromatherapy can be used in several ways from lighting a candle, applying to pressure points, spritzing on a pillow or adding to a hot bath. For example, basil is used for migraines while lavender is used as an anti-inflammatory.

8. *Hypnotherapy*: Hypnotherapy is a skilled verbal communication which helps direct a client's imagination in such a way as to bring about intended alterations in sensations, perceptions, feelings, thoughts and behavior (National Hypnotherapy Society). Hypnotherapy has been known to be successfully used during childbirth to help women manage pain during labor. Hypnotherapy can be self-taught or implemented from a trained therapist.

9. *Yoga*: yoga or simple stretching are simple practices that should be applied to everyday life to reduce the tension of stress and keep the muscles in proper working order. There are specific stretches that can focus on problem areas such as the neck or lower back. These stretches can be assigned from a personal trainer, massage therapist or physiotherapist. Yoga can be enjoyed at home or in a studio with several other participants. There are many forms of yoga ranging from hatha yoga to hot yoga. The focus in yoga is on breath control, meditation, stretching and balance. Not all forms of yoga are spiritual with chants and mantras if you don't feel comfortable with that form of practice.

Chapter 5

What aggravates pain?

Several studies and researches have been conducted, but until now, researchers are still clueless as to the things that aggravate pain. It was discovered, however, that the things which can alleviate pain are also the same things that can aggravate it. Furthermore, according to their studies, people generally do not know what exactly are the things or factors that can alleviate or aggravate their pain. Here are several factors:

1. *Activity*: Activity can aggravate the pain and worsen the situation. For example, a person who sprained his ankle is not allowed to move freely without a cane or support. If he uses his feet without support, the sprained ankle will have to carry the full weight thus, applying pressure on the injured ankle will make it worse and walking will be more painful. Changing positions can also aggravate pain because it adds pressure and force on the injured area.

2. *Foods and Oral Activities*: Eating is sometimes helpful, but oftentimes, it aggravates pain as well. When the person is sick, it is best to give him soft foods like mashed potatoes or porridge. In some situations however, even soft foods are still painful. Just the act of opening the mouth is already painful in some situations. Chewing is not advisable for tooth aches and during post dental surgeries. Intake of acidic foods and liquids is also prohibited, especially in the case of ulcer and canker sores. Kissing or talking is equally painful when the lip is busted or when there's a wound in the mouth. Furthermore, certain foods can cause adverse reactions in the body. For example, acidic type foods can exasperate arthritis symptoms. Gluten and milk products are known to elevate symptoms in the body causing inflammation.

3. *Inactivity*: As much as activity aggravates pain, inactivity can also aggravate it. Inactivity causes blood circulation to be stagnant and it produces pain. It produces a numbing pain when you sit for long period of time. If you are hospitalized and your position is unchanged for several days, you will develop bed sores and it's painful.

4. *Stress*: Stress also is a contributing factor that aggravates pain. Stress is known to be the "silent killer." When the body perceives a threat, it enters into a "fight or flight" response. When we are prepared to "fight", the adrenaline in our body increases and the cortisol hormone rises. This is normal and usually drops off when the stress is dealt with. However, if a person is in constant stress and has an overexposure to cortisol in the body, their health is quick to deteriorate and the body's healing process is ruptured. Sleeplessness also impedes the immune system from working properly thus, inflammation and swelling becomes worse. A fresh wound can also start to bleed and may reopen if a person is emotionally unstable, angry, or depressed.

5. *Medical Treatment*: As much as medical treatment can alleviate and relieve pain altogether, it can also make it worse. There are medications which produce harmful and painful side effects to the person being treated. For example, aspirins; they are indeed pain relievers and very powerful at that, however, when taken on a daily basis, it destroys gastrointestinal lining causing painful spasms and acute pain in the stomach. Chemotherapy is also another factor which aggravates pain, as well as surgery.

6. *Touch/Applications*: In severe physical injuries, pressure is needed to stop the bleeding. There are times however, when touching the injured area is not very advisable. This is true with those injured in motor or vehicular accidents. One wrong touch on the affected area can kill the person or

worsen the injury. There may be broken bones which are better left untouched and without pressure. Similarly, if the affected area is already infected and swelling is really severe, touching it becomes unbearably painful. This is the case of burn victims. The skin or the flesh is open and touching it is ultimately the most painful thing that they will hope never to experience. Antiseptic or cleaning their wound will make them cry in pain that is incomparable to anything else.

7. *Temperature* - Temperature can also aggravate the pain. This is most often the case for older people. Arthritis and other joint problems are at their most painful during the winter season. Bone cancer patients are most susceptible to severe pain during the cold season. Skin problems on the other hand, are most painful during the hot season or summer when the skin becomes dry. This is most particularly true when perspiration seeps into the wound.

8. *Posture* - Poor posture can also exasperate the pain, especially for people who suffer back and neck pain. Slouching, sitting too long, standing with one hip jutting out, twisting the body, improper lifting, crossing legs, or caring a backpack on one shoulder are many of the ways that our bodies can be thrown out of alignment. It is important to get up and stretch when sitting in a chair or car for too long. Every couple hours is recommended. When watching television, face the screen head on rather than twisting your body to view the screen. Practice sitting up right when at the computer or using electronic devises. It is best to not keep your head in the down position for too long. Movement is the key to keeping muscles loose in the body.

9. *Toxins* - environmental toxins can contribute to inflammation in the body and elevate the chronic pain. Toxins can include air quality, heavy metals in food or

materials, pesticides, chemical fertilizers, antibiotics and hormones in food products, genetically modified foods, plastic containers, and nitrates in deli meats, artificial coloring/flavors/sweeteners, and chemical detergents. The list is endless. Eliminating or reducing these toxins in your environment is crucial. People even go another step further and partake in routine detoxes and cleanses to rid the body of these harmful toxins.

Chapter 6

How to Prevent Relapses

A relapse is that part of the recovery process when a person may tend to go back to his ineffective pain management ways, giving rise to yet another round of pain. It is a common symptom that may be brought about by drug or medical dependency inherent to two-thirds of the patients who have experienced chronic pain despite their intention not to do so. Having said that, relapse is more properly defined as a progressive series of events that takes someone away from stable recovery to a state of becoming dysfunctional in their current recovery.

There are several ways on how people who have recovered can prevent painful relapses:

1. *Do Not Overwork Yourself*: It is natural that the body will feel so much better and stronger after a series of treatments. In chronic pain, it is logical that people with this condition know what things trigger their physical pain the most. To prevent the pain in coming back again and persisting for longer periods of time, the person should not overwork himself. He should still rest until completely recovered. Only then can he or she be able to sustain full recovery.

2. *Stay Rested and Have a Good Sleep*: Nothing is better than a good night's sleep to detoxify and cleanse the body. Sleep helps in repairing tissues and corroded cells. If you sleep at night and you are well-rested, your body will be able to recuperate faster.

3. *Relapse Education*: This is the most vital stage in relapse prevention. The relapser needs to be educated. He needs to

understand that what he is going through is a normal stage in the process of recovery and that there is something he can do to overcome it. The person needs to be sober from drugs or any medication for him to understand it.

4. *Live a Balanced Life*: The relapser, once educated and if he properly understands what he is going through, will be able to recognize warning signs or problems that trigger the relapse. He can create a list of his own personal warning signs or reasons why. This way, he can do something about the triggers and prevent them from happening. For example, she may notice that when she does certain activities or eats certain foods, relapse is initiated. Living a balanced diet and life should be prioritized to experience pain-free existence.

Chapter 7

Understanding TMS

What is TMS?

The condition is given the name Tension Myositis Syndrome (TMS) by Dr. John E. Sarno. It has also been called Tension Myoneural Syndrome and lately, the Mind-Body Syndrome. According to its descriptions, the condition is characterized by psyche-generated or psychogenic nerve and musculoskeletal symptoms, one of the most common being back pain.

Dr. Sarno, who has written about Tension Myositis Syndrome in four of his books, spoke of the condition being involved in other disorders that features pain as well. The protocol for TMS treatment includes writing about the patients' emotional issues, education about the condition, and resumption of their normal lifestyle, with or without supporting counseling sessions or psychotherapy. These treatments are found to be very effective for treatment of psychosomatic symptoms that results in chronic pain. Statistically, TMS treatments are also found to have outperformed other treatments targeting the same symptoms with a different approach than that forwarded by Dr. Sarno.

Symptoms and Diagnosis

Tension myositis syndrome has always been associated with chronic back pains; but many more types and locations of the pain are found to have been caused by the condition.

TMS symptoms may include either individual experience or in a combination of the following:

23

- Pain
- Weakness
- Numbness
- Stiffness
- Tingling
- Dermatological disorder
- Gastrointestinal problems
- Repetitive-strain injury

Although occurring most frequently as localized back pains, tension myoneural syndrome can also manifest on other parts of the body. It may be on the wrists, arms, knees or neck. It has also been found that the symptoms have a tendency to move around the body. It is a significant indicator that if the symptoms move locations during treatment, that the pain is from TMS.

Sarno and Schechter have proposed a list of criterion for the diagnosis of TMS:

- *A History of Other Psychosomatic Disorders*

  Tension headaches, irritable bowel movement and other psychosomatic disorders experienced in the past may be an indication that an individual is suffering from tension myositis syndrome.

- *The Lack of a Definite Physical Cause for the Symptoms*

  A completed physical examination and other imaging studies would be able to rule out the influence of any other serious physical conditions. For example, the herniation on the spinal discs is usually blamed for pain and numbness in certain areas, even if the herniation location is not correlated with the location of the symptom.

- *Tender Points*

  Medical doctors often use tender points in certain key areas in the body to pinpoint the affliction and the cause of the symptoms. In 99% of TMS-diagnosed patients, eight tender points are often seen: two tender points in the lateral upper buttocks, two in the lumbar paraspinal muscles and two more points in the upper trapezius muscles.

It is highly recommended for patients who think they have TMS to visit a traditional medical doctor first. That is to be able to fully ascertain that the symptoms are not from any underlying physical disorders.

Treatments

Treatment for tension myositis syndrome is a protocol that includes proper education about the patient's condition, writing and contemplation about their emotional issues and finally, a resumption of their normal lifestyle. For patients that are not responding that much to the regular treatment, additional support is given through counseling sessions and possibly, psychotherapy.

- *Education about TMS*

  This may take form in various modes of media. It may be through lectures, visitations or reference materials such as texts and audio content. The education would cover both physiological and psychological aspects of the disorder. This would allow their patients to learn that their physical condition is actually normal, and that any pain and disability they have is actually a result of deconditioning, fear of the recurrence of pain and experiencing the same injury again.

- *Writing about their Emotional Issues*

Specialists in tension myoneural syndrome attribute the disorder's symptoms to repressed emotions and fears. In such situations, the best solution is an awareness of these emotions. By facing the repressed fears head-on, individuals suffering from TMS symptoms defeat the repression through constant practice of meditation techniques and daily psychological processing.

With this in mind, the patients going through TMS treatment are given two writing assignments that they have to continuously repeat over a period of time. It is to list down all the issues that may contribute to their repressed emotions. These include their personality traits, the current pressures in their life, their childhood traumas and experiences, as well as issues of mortality and aging. This would generally include situations and experiences where the patient represses anger and other negative emotions, consciously or otherwise. Their next assignment is to write down in-depth essays about each of the items in their list. By writing longer on each item that they have identified, the patient is forced to look at the issues closely and possibly find resolution for them. Even if they don't do so, it would still be beneficial for the treatment. Here, the patient themselves come to have more insight regarding their own issues. It is found to be more therapeutic rather than someone else giving their own opinions on the said issues.

- *Resumption of the Patient's Normal Lifestyle*

There are two steps to this part of the patient's treatment. Firstly, all regular physical activity is resumed. The patients are recommended to become gradually active and slowly return to their normal life. They are also encouraged to get rid of habits previously obtained as safety behaviors meant to protect their "damaged" area – the location of the symptoms. The second part to this step is to discontinue treatments like physical therapy and spinal manipulation. As the patient is properly diagnosed with tension myositis syndrome, any physical treatment that were meant for disorders caused by other physical disorders will only reinforce the erroneous structural "root" of pain and other symptoms.

- *Meetings for Support and Counseling*

For patients who have problems responding to the previous steps of the treatment for TMS, additional support meetings may be arranged. There they may receive help with exploring their emotional issues; they can also review their education to get more clarification to further enhance their knowledge of their condition.

- *Recovery Program and Psychotherapy*

For the patients who do not make prompt recovery upon completion of the treatment, extensions or repetition of the treatment is coupled with six to ten sessions of psychotherapy. It is considered to be an option only for the few serious cases that show almost no response to the treatments, this method uses analytically-oriented dynamic psychotherapy.

There are also recovery programs available, packaged into audio and video sessions that are specially designed to cover the therapeutic concepts. The articles, segments and exercises are made to exemplify the healing process thus starting the treatment for the condition.

Studies, Theory and Controversy

Tension myositis syndrome is a more controversial modality than pain disorder and psychogenic pain, both of which are now accepted diagnoses in the community of medicine. Multiple studies have already been made to attest the effectiveness of the treatments associated with TMS.

Researchers have stated that there is an advantage in the way that TMS treatments don't recommend medicine prescriptions and surgical procedures; it avoids the many risks. But since the disorder is relatively new, and the patients having been diagnosed and treated for it are still relatively low in number, any risk of the treatment is unknown.

The theory behind TMS, according to Dr. Sarno, is that the condition is initiated by unconscious emotional issues causing the symptoms, most particularly the manifestation of pain. It is suggested that, by using the autonomic nervous system, the unconscious mind decreases blood flow to certain areas of the body such as tendons, muscles and nerves that results to oxygen deprivation. This will then manifest as pain in the tissues affected. The most prominent characteristic to this condition is the migration of the pained area up and down the spine or from side to side. This movement implies that the pain may not be caused by any injury or physical deformity.

The theory then states that as a defense mechanism, the patient's mind uses the pain as a distraction from unconscious negative emotions and mental stress. This could be unconscious anxiety, anger and narcissistic rage. As the conscious mind is distracted by the pain, this type of psychological repression prevents the negative emotions from spilling out, keeping it tightly in the unconscious mind instead.

Dr. Sarno has always been a critic of conventional medicine diagnoses regarding back pain. As the usual treatments for them are rest, exercise, and physical therapy – with or without the surgery – they usually reinforce the emotional repression, and restrict the pain into the physical awareness.

The diagnosis and treatment for tension myoneural syndrome are not accepted to the majority of the medical community. But although mainstream medicine does not accept it, there are many notable doctors who do include TMS in the possible causes of localized pains and recommend TMS treatment for them.

The controversy of TMS as a theory and the effectiveness of its treatment reside in the fact that it hasn't been proven in a clinical trial that has been properly controlled. This quality is an inherent difficulty in conducting clinical trials for all psychosomatic illnesses such as TMS. Critics attribute its massive success rate into "placebo effect" and "regression to the mean" as there is only a small number of cases that are diagnosed and treated. It is also attributed to the fact that most cases of back pain resolve themselves within a few weeks. This is countered by TMS treatment doctors by responding that their successfully recovered patients are those who have approached and have been treated by them only after exhausting all other possibility of any underlying physical or psychological disorder in mainstream medicine. And that these people relied on them as a last resort. Indeed, it is highly recommended by TMS doctors to be completely sure that there are no underlying physical causes for their condition, with the proof subject to their evaluation.

Other Important Notes about TMS

Here are some other suggestions with this book's very own commentaries that are from various resources that deal with tension myositis syndrome:

- *Your Own Inner Witness*

In many TMS materials, experiences in the past where the individual experiences negative emotions can cause trouble and pain later on. Usually, people are able to express their emotions fluently as normal. And then after a period of time, they would just stop and move on from the issue; that is, even if their mind is still not ready for the recovery. This would result in a repressed emotion that will stay in the unconscious. When triggered or pressured, these will manifest into physical pain and other conditions like skin disorders and gastrointestinal anxiety to distract the mind away from emotional and psychological stress.

- *Nobody is Perfect*

One of the most common psychological stresses that causes tension myoneural syndrome is the daily demand for a person to work harder, to be good, to please everyone, to succeed; in short, to be perfect. The pain is made by the mind to distract the self from the rising anger of being unable to be so, and not wanting to answer to these demands. This conflict can be resolved by the realization of this issue, combined with self-acceptance and contentment exercises – counting what you have, opposed to focusing on what you don't, celebrating what you've achieved rather than looking back on what you failed upon – that will help ease the pressure you have placed on yourself.

- *Reflection is One of Your Best Weapons*

One of the major steps in the treatment of the mind-body syndrome is to write down your issues and contemplate on them. One has to practice reflection as often as they can for this to work. It is usually hard for individuals to reflect deeper and delve into their unconscious issues. That is because these are usually conglomerations of many factors that includes their entire emotional history, their personality traits, their current issues in life, as well as how they view the world and how they think the world views them. The key to reflection is to discard the fear of seeing something in yourself that you do not like. The more you shy away from the unpleasant facets of yourself, the more your unconscious will bury the important things away from your awareness.

- *Placebo Effectiveness*

Many who are aware that their pain has come from psychosomatic roots may have tried placebo treatments. Critics actually attribute the success of TMS treatments to the placebo effect. The only problem lies on the possibility of repeat episodes of the disorder after such a method. Time and time again, it has been proven that the human mind is a wonderful thing able to do such amazing feats. And this is the root of the placebo effect. Placebo treatments rely on the patient's complete belief that they are being treated, so their mind therefore, will treat the body accordingly. Just like how humans, by habit and conditioning, have learned to feel hungry at certain times in a day. That is, although humans can survive ingesting sustenance only once a day, or every few days for that matter, they have learned to "need" three full meals in daily. Although TMS treatment is not entirely in the placebo category, it does utilize the great power of the mind to heal itself.

- *Growing your Own Pain*

Once a certain negative emotion takes root in your unconscious, you naturally stack them up over time. The mind is a very organized being, no matter how chaotic you think your thought processes are. Human minds tend to categorize things and stack similar thoughts together. This naturally applies to the unconscious mind as well. This is the very reason why you can recall other instances that made you cry when you start crying. The mind links one memory with others that have the same emotional pull or significance. That is to say, unconscious anger will continue to build up as long as you are not aware of it enough to vent it. And soon, it will be causing unnecessary tension that will manifest into TMS pain and symptoms. One way to avoid this is to deal with an emotion as soon as they are formed. It may be awkward at first, but it will surely help in the long run. Get mad when you're angry, cry when you feel like doing so and vent all the bad things out whenever you can. If you can resolve the smaller issues just when they come into being, the faster you will be able to truly move on from them. That is, to avoid keeping them in, to be dealt in at a more "appropriate" time. There is no such thing, if you feel it now, deal with it now. It will save you from further self-incrimination in the future.

- *Awareness of your Habits and Behavioral Patterns*

Some people may react to stress by turning in to themselves. They tighten their face and head muscles which will definitely result in a headache later on. Others dilate or constrict blood vessels that limit the blood flow and therefore deprive certain body parts from much needed oxygen. Pain would then be experienced, including migraines and other localized pains because of this. The habits may not be observable easily, but with proper diagnosis and monitoring, these stress reactions can be removed by habitually practicing a conscious relaxation from the tension. Identifying when exactly that is may be difficult, since it would have been ingrained so deep into the person's habit that it would be indistinguishable from other involuntary body activity. For this, there are devices that can be requested to be used – called biofeedback – that will tell you when your body keeps on regressing into tension. A woman who had a case of temporo-mandibular disorder was found to have the habit of tensing her neck and jaws when she's stressed. Trying out the biofeedback device, the electronic box almost constantly lighted up, telling her that she's doing "it" again. After relaxation practice, which took some time getting used to, she's able to remove her habit and is now pain-free.

- *Overcoming Safety Behaviors, Awareness*

Usually when people experience pain, they tend to rely on deeply ingrained medical teachings on how to "take care" of one's body while it is "damaged". This usually involves avoiding certain physical activities that are deemed to be too strenuous and might have even caused the damage before. Because of this, lifestyles may be hindered and normal life is interrupted. It is as if time has come to a stagnant stop until the pain goes away, so that you can go back to what you were doing before. But the pain doesn't go; so you wait more, doing next to nothing. If you are diagnosed with TMS, you have to get rid of that habit of treating yourself as if you're breakable. The thought that you are fragile in your condition, and the fear that one wrong movement will cause pain, make up for a huge reinforcement to your stress. These in turn, will cause more pain.

- *Triggers*

Once you have identified your key issues that are the source of your TMS syndromes, you should also be able to see exactly what triggers reactions to these emotions. Subtle reminders from both the environment and your thought processes my trigger pain relapses. If you can pinpoint these triggers, you can analyze why exactly you are linking them to previously experienced issues. This way, you are processing more and more of the emotional impacts of your experiences. Awareness is one of the key features used in tension myositis syndrome treatment. The more you know, the more you are able to sort out the issues from within themselves. Doing so will make the inherent repression useless and the physical pain distraction to be unnecessary.

- *Understanding to Heal*

Healing psychosomatic disorders such as TMS basically requires a combination of understanding your condition, the reason why it came to be and a sort of constant self-reflection. Internal conflicts are usually the root of psychosomatic disorders. Resolving those conflict will ease up the pressure that the resulting stress has caused, leading into a gradual self-healing.

One of the things you have to understand is that there are a large number of people who are also experiencing the same things you are. That they are also suffering from the same pain you do even if it is in a different intensity in a different body part. You are not alone and you are not prohibited from asking help. Connecting with people who are going through the same things you are is a good way to slowly accept your condition. None of the treatments can ever help you if you do not accept that you are suffering from the condition in the first place. Many people have difficulties in doing so, preferring to blame it on a physical injury or disorder, on something that they can take a pill or have a surgery for. The fear of facing one's self and acknowledging that the problem is within you is one of the biggest hurdles that a TMS sufferer has to face. But it is not so much of a bother to those who have gone through almost all physical treatments, as they have already realized that the problem is not with their body but in their mind. That is why those who have gone through various physical therapies and such in the past respond more favorably to TMS treatments than those who have resorted to it earlier.

- *Personalities and Low Self-Esteem Causing Pain*

  Certain personality traits like being a perfectionist or a pessimist can result to the manifestation of tension myositis syndrome. The compulsive, nearly obsessive preoccupation with perfecting everything and the fear of failure, as well as thoughts of things going wrong can put quite a strain on a person's psyche. The pressure can then be repressed through the unconscious mind by distracting the self with psychosomatic physical pains. And because these are personality traits that are formed over a person's lifetime, it is harder to identify and even more difficult to change.

  Low self-esteem is also a leading cause of TMS symptoms. It causes a person to be very cautious in their every move and generally too careful with their dealings with others. As the pessimistic-version of the urge for perfection is amplified, the more the unconscious mind might be strained to the point of transferring the pressure into a physical distraction, as mentioned before.

- *Rage and Withholding Anger*

  Withholding anger, most especially explosive rage, puts a massive pressure on the unconscious mind. Consciously swallowing your anger can be very destructive, turning your violent thoughts inward, causing stress for your emotions. Also, not letting anyone know of your emotional upheaval does not resolve the root. The rage would just simmer and be very sensitive. Flicking towards the boiling point over every little trigger-reminder you encounter.

Lately, this has seen many solutions. With the advent of internet and anonymous social media, one can freely express their anger, flinging it into the universe instead of keeping it in. Of course, there are still a lot of people who have made turning anger inwards a habit. For these people, they should have a way to vent their anger and frustration to ease the emotional stress that such feelings bring onto their own mind.

This could be in a form of a journal or diary, where the person can just write down everything that is going through their mind. There is actually a case where a teenage girl suffering from constant chest aches and "heavy feelings", has never been attributed to any existing physical cause. After discovering that she has a habit of not speaking at their school, she is made to keep a "Poison Notebook" where she writes down all the bad things she kept on thinking about other people. After a month of doing so, she returned to her sessions reporting the loss of her chest aches and a general decline in the "viciousness" of her thoughts. The counselor was presented her notebook and it was marked that, after a few weeks of endless notes dripping pure vitriol, her thought-notes have become less malign.

For other people, physical "violence" is the best way to vent anger. Hitting pillows, punching sandbags and such actions can help them fizzle out their rage. There is actually this one organization that has a "Rage Wall". People can come to their place filled with plates, cups, glasses, vases, pots and even appliances like old, unused TVs and radios. The visitors can then just keep on grabbing the items and throw them at the wall decorated with speech bubbles saying, "I hate you!" "Go fall in a ditch and die!" "Damn you!" and other angry lines that people can aim their plate – or cup, or TV – at. There is only one rule in the place. Don't hit anyone, just the walls.

- *Highly Sensitive People and those with Too Much Need for Attention*

These kinds of people generally think they are very fragile. And a deep-seated thought like that could make the notion a reality. These traits are usually a leftover characteristic from a previous experience that can date back to their childhood years. They tend to over-analyze things and overthink every little comment directed at them. This habit can create imaginary stress on a person's mind that can result in emotional pressures that are very real, leading up to a TMS-prone constitution.

- *Depression, Fatigue and Anxiety*

Depression, fatigue and anxiety can be very stressing to handle for the mind. Being unable to relax for long periods of time can hurt a person's unconscious mind. One of the traits common to these three, is the inability to share their condition with anyone. It could be because of situational circumstances or a disinclination to do so. Because of the heightened stress on the psyche, coupled with the weakening of the physical, these can contribute to the appearance of TMS symptoms such as migraines and body pain.

- *Drugs and Pain*

Many psychosomatic disorders that feature pain as a symptom are wrongfully diagnosed as other physical illness. These people are then prescribed with pain medication. Now, since pain-reducing medicine target the actual area of the affliction – for example, the lower back – they are unable to ease the pain. Why? That is because the symptom is induced straight at the part of the brain dealing with the feeling of pain. And since the prescription does not help with the pain, the dosage or the medication strength is increased, with the same result. They end up desensitizing the body from the pain medication, rendering them ineffective at the instances that they are truly needed. Not only that, but you are also endangering the function of your organs that receive the stress of continuously ingesting the medication. The building up of the substances in your body may cause trouble in the near future.

- *Healing Yourself*

In all psychosomatic disorders such as tension myositis syndrome, self-healing is the most important facet of the treatment. Some people may prefer to let someone – usually their doctor – to boss them around, to tell them what to do and what not to do, what to eat, what they can't. This way the blame is on the physician when the treatment doesn't succeed. This should be changed. Even with conventional physical treatments, one should lord over themselves. This means accepting the healing and telling their body to recover. Without the will and determination to be healed, treatments would be just that – treatments – and not solutions.

- *Visualization and Setting Goals*

In connection to healing oneself, visualization and setting goals are important. You should have one big goal – to fully heal and return to normal, or an even better life – and some small milestones you will set for yourself. Visualizing a life where you are pain-less and is free to do whatever you want can help in cementing your determination to heal. This will also keep you up when the emotionally-taxing treatment brings you a bit down. By setting a final goal at the end of smaller goals, the big one feels easier. This is achieved by slowly traversing through the smaller goals one by one. Set a daily or weekly goal and visualize what you will be able to think and do by the end of that time period.

Always give yourself some time to feel the celebration of your accomplishment for every milestone. Not only will it give you a needed break in your climb towards betterment, you will also feel more encouraged to go on and reach the final goal.

- *Communication*

Communication is very important in all treatments, most especially for psychosomatic conditions. Firstly, that should be with your doctor or counselor. Making regular updates with your progress can help them assess any need for adjustment and can also encourage you when you are hesitating in stepping onward. Communicating with your friends and family can provide immense amounts of support. Psychosomatic treatments can be very trying for relationships, but the best ones weather through by constant support and understanding. You'll come out of the experience together even closer and tighter than before. Also, communicating with other people suffering the same conditions as you do can be quite a help. With the internet and other forms of communication, it would be easy to get connected with these people. It is still quite a different kind of support to give and receive encouragements from people who are experiencing the same things as you do. The feeling of helping others out is also quite a good addition to your self-healing.

- *Mindful Meditation*

Many relaxation techniques and meditation exercises can be combined with an ongoing TMS treatment. By meditating, the patient can better explore their psyche and emotions as well as relaxing the body to let go of the involuntary tensions. These usually cause the pain and fatigue that are characteristic to psychosomatic disorders. Chronic pain sufferers tend to think "this will go on forever", "I'll never get better" or "I'm no good for anything anymore." By meditating on the positives and encouraging oneself, such hurdles are crossed and stresses are released, readying the mind and body for the healing to set in.

- *Laughter*

As always, laughter is still the best medicine. Induced feeling of happiness or even generally feeling good can do wonders for your condition. Doing fun things, watching funny movies and shows, or even just finding something to laugh at, helps you get over your negative emotions. Have fun with your friends and family. Enjoy hilarity wherever you can find them. Look into the brighter side of things. Soon enough, you'll be laughing at your previous worries like a wise man (or woman).

- *Comfort your Enemy*

In these treatments, your worst enemy is yourself. It is observed that people are generally more able to give advice and think of solutions for problems and anxieties of other people. So think of your own situations objectively. Comfort and give advice to yourself as if you're helping your best friend, or a close family. You are your greatest friend and your closest family after all; just as you are your worst enemy. It works both ways, you know. Of course, such an activity that requires clarity of thought and focus of your mind requires that you, yourself has identified what exactly is wrong. So dig in and help that pain-filled, trembling you inside that darkened interior of your heart.

- *Letting Go*

There are root-causes for TMS that cannot be resolved either because they are entirely out of your control or because they are in the past and long gone. It is very painful to blame yourself for something that you have no control over. It has been one of the leading causes for TMS symptoms and are usually either self-imposed or are drilled into them all throughout a significant period of time. It could also be an experience long gone in the past that no one can do anything about anymore. In such cases, letting go would be the best option. One cannot totally forget memories, especially those that are heavy enough to cause impacts that affect you physically in the present. But they can be accepted, acknowledged and regarded as valuable stepping stones for the current you to reach where you are now. Don't endanger the future for something that happened in the past. Let them be your inspiration, your motivation to keep moving forward and up, instead of taking them with you like shackles that remind you of the pain. Don't live in the past, gradually move on into the present and be hopeful for your future.

These notes can be treated more like a points-to-ponder for your TMS education. This is an integral part of the treatment towards a pain-free lifestyle. Complete peace and contentment with your own body and life may be impossible, but striving towards it – without stressing yourself; never that, it's counterproductive – is a good course to follow.

Conclusion

Thank you again for purchasing this book!

I hope this book was able to help you understand what pain is and how our body responds to painful stimulus. Furthermore, the objective of this book is to help you become aware of the negative effects pain can bring into your life and how you will be able to cope with it. There are several factors which can alleviate and aggravate pain and surely, you are already knowledgeable about those things. The next step is to apply this learning and share these helpful tips and information to other people, especially to those who are currently undergoing painful recovery.

Always remember that pain is only temporary. It goes away after the wound is healed. You have to accept that pain is a part of life and it is normal to be hurt sometimes. Do not succumb to the depressing stage of that painful experience. Pain is inevitable, but suffering is optional. Learn how to be strong and cope with pain accordingly. Do not suppress yourself. Share your pain with your loved ones because if pain is shared, it becomes more bearable. Never try to carry it all by yourself. After all, there really is no name for the pain.

Be hungry for the pain free life you deserve. Don't stop till you achieve relief from your symptoms. Dig deep to find the root causes and dig them out of your life. Keep persevering until you find the results you are looking for. Don't settle for status quo...you are worth much more than that. Your body is designed to be healthy and to live life to its fullest. Have hope for a future that is pain free.

Finally, if you enjoyed this book and found it meaningful, please take the time to share your thoughts and *post a positive review* on Amazon. I greatly appreciate your time and effort.

I would love for you to share your experiences, stories and encouragements with me. My email address is *miasoleilkindle@gmail.com*.

In addition, please remember to check out our Facebook page in order to find other resources and upcoming promotions:

https://www.facebook.com/joypublishing

Thank you, from the bottom of my heart and I wish you the best.

With gratitude,

Mia Soleil

One Last Thing...

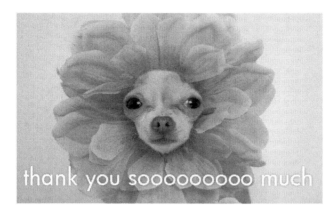

Source: Wikipedia

If you believe that this book is worth sharing, would you please take the time to let others know how it affected your life? If it turns out to make a difference in the lives of others, they will be forever grateful to you, as will I.

Made in the USA
San Bernardino, CA
25 February 2017